Praises for Heal My PCOS and Melissa Madgwick

After only 1 month I don't have any cysts on my ovaries anymore and Mel I have you and your book to thank for that. If it wasn't for you I don't think I would have got back to normal. Now I finally believe I have a chance at getting pregnant. I no longer get bloated when I have a period. I no longer crave sugar. I truly hope every woman buys your book. I can never thank you enough for all your help. In such a short time I've seen huge differences. Even my hubby says thank you.

- Amanda Humphries

After reading your book on Amazon 10 months ago I had some hope. I was told by medical professionals that I wouldn't be able to fall pregnant easily or at all due to my PCOS. Now thanks to this book, I am four months pregnant with my first child and have never felt better. Thank you for being an inspiration.

- Jade James

Thank you for your book Melissa. I wanted to let you know that I'm doing well and I'm still implementing all that I've learnt from your book. I'm making an effort to remain positive and not give in to any negative thoughts. I just thought it would be nice to let you know that there have been very good changes ever since I read your book. Thank you so much once again.

- P.Naik

Heal my PCOS

**MELISSA MADGWICK, BA
CERTIFIED HEALTH COACH**

CONSCIOUS CARE PUBLISHING PTY LTD

HEAL MY PCOS
Your Journey to Healing from Polycycstic Ovarian Syndrome Naturally

First Published 2016 by: Conscious Care Publishing Pty Ltd
33 Crompton Road, Rockingham, WA 6168, Australia
PO Box 776, Rockingham, WA 6968, Australia
Phone: (61+) 1300 814 115   www.consciouscarepublishing.com.au

First Edition printed November 2016.

National Library of Australia Cataloguing-in-Publication entry:
Author: Madgwick, Melissa, 1985-
Heal my PCOS / by Melissa Madgwick
ISBN 9780994540461 (Paperback), 9780994540478 (Digital)
Brand Dominance Pty Ltd, Cover Illustrator.
Hudson, Rocky, Editor.
Hannah Laidlaw, Photographer.

Printed by Lightning Source
Typeset & cover design by Conscious Care Publishing Pty Ltd

618.11

ISBN: 978-0-9945404-6-1

To Lilly

This book was written with the love, strength and guidance from my beautiful Lilly. Thank you for all the lessons taught and happiness brought into my life's journey.

I will always remember your warmth and energy. I know from the depths of my soul we will meet again. However, until then, you'll forever be in my heart. I love you.

Contents

Acknowledgements

I'd like to thank some special people in my life, who have crossed my path over the many years and have inspire me to keep growing as a person.

To my partner Andrew, I love you with all my soul. Thank you for believing in me and pushing me to get this book out there to reach and inspire women with my story.

You are my rock, my light and my You'll never realise the positive impact you've had on my life. I'm blessed to have met you again in this lifetime. I love you.

To my mum and dad, thank you for you cheering me on from the sidelines and teaching me there is no limit in life. I have learnt so many grateful lessons from you both.

To my sister, thank you for your love and I'll always remember our innocence.

To my team at Brand Dominance, thank you for your endless hours of putting together the design elements for this book. Your talents, enthusiasm and gorgeous energies me make excited to wake up each morning to work on great projects together and help businesses across the globe be seen in heard in their respective marketplaces through branding, design and marketing.

A big thank you to Liz, my publisher and guide. I'm so appreciative for your confidence in this book and helping me publish my first book! I'm forever thankful for assisting this gigantic dream of mine become real.

And lastly, a big thank you to all the beautiful women who have reached out to me with your vulnerable PCOS stories over the past three years. My heart sings every time I hear a small win and/or step closer to your own recovery.

Many of you have kept this book alive with your appreciation, love and feedback. Keep making positive changes in your own life, and thus educating and inspiring others with your newfound information learnt. This book is for you.

Forward

Before doing anything you read in this book, speak with your health professional about your ideas. Craft a plan together as you move forward. Your health professional knows you.

I have not attended medical school. I have not been licensed by any kind of committee or board or government to give any health advice.

I have found, however, that most medical doctors have lost sight of the fact that food can be medicine, that humans are not inherently broken and that diseases can be cured by simple, healthful life choices.

I have read hundreds of blogs, and poured many hours of research into the journey of healing myself, naturally.

You are the captain of your own body and health, and I advise you to weigh my words, your doctor's words and everything you read against your own experience, instincts and knowledge.

With my love and light. This is for you.

Five Reasons to Read This Book

#1 Learn from my success story

This book is full of my experiences, failures, learning and successes during my recovery from PCOS. My goal is that I want women to know how to heal themselves naturally from this syndrome.

I would like to open your eyes to the diversity of polycystic ovarian syndrome as well as showing you there are easy and natural interventions for overcoming it. Feel empowered with the information in this book. I've broken it down with stories, simple tips and advice to make it easy to follow. Give a woman a prescription and she may find relief for a few weeks. Give a woman a book and she will heal herself permanently. This could be the best few dollars you have ever spent.

#2 You are not alone

If you've been diagnosed with PCOS, you probably feel like you've reached a dead end: alone and an outcast from 'real life'. But please know, you're not on your own! At least 1 in 10 women are diagnosed with PCOS during their lives, and EVERY DAY 10% of women aged between 12 and 45 are told "You have PCOS". There is hope! You can get your life back as I and many other women have.

#3 Know your cause

I discuss the four main types of PCOS – what they are and how to manage each. Every woman is different. PCOS is the root effect of SOMETHING being thrown off in your body - largely due to what you are eating, thinking and/or how you treat yourself. The tools that helped me and countless other women are in my book. You CAN heal your PCOS symptoms and get your life back again. The only way to heal PCOS and its associated symptoms is to get at the underlying cause of the hormonal imbalance. Sure, weight can be a factor. In fact, 50% of women with the syndrome are overweight. But while many believe weight to be a contributing factor, it's a symptom, not the cause of the problem as many women with PCOS are not considered to be overweight. You can take charge today!

#4 Learn the best diet and supplements for PCOS

Women suffering with PCOS tend to be deficient in a number of key vitamins and other nutrients, so they need the right food and nutrition. Supplements will complement your diet and accelerate its impact on rebalancing your hormones. You'll learn all about my low-GI PCOS eating plan and easy-to-follow supplement guide. You can then shop for, prepare and enjoy eating real food. You'll be surprised how different you feel after you take this advice!

#5 Over 50 tips and tricks on how I healed

In this book, there are multiple tips and tricks on how I healed myself naturally which will not cost the earth. There are countless other women's stories as well. Your doctor may prescribe medication that covers up symptoms in the short term. One prescription may cost $25, $50, $75 or even $100. And that may last you just a few months.

Heal My PCOS will last you for the rest of your life!

Free book resources page

Some of the content couldn't fit in these pages, so I have collated all in a free book resources page!

Visit: www.healmypcos.com/resources to download:

- Simple to follow eating suggestions
- Supplements recommendations
- Must have foods in your kitchen
- Diagrams and flow charts of the types of PCOS
- Five ways to beat PCOS today
- Real-life testimonials
- And more...

Join the conversation as you read

Email: info@healmypcos.com

Website: www.healmypcos.com

Twitter: www.twitter.com/healmypcos

Facebook: www.facebook.com/healmypcos

You are not alone

If you have polycystic ovarian syndrome, you are one of millions of women in the Western World who suffer from it. Up to 10% of women between 12 and 45 acquire PCOS, and it is considered by some to be the leading cause of infertility. Yes, you can get your life back!

You may have been told there is no cure. By "cure," the medical community means a patented pharmaceutical to address the symptoms. And it's a good thing they haven't. The real cure for PCOS is to change the behaviors, eating habits and lifestyle choices that caused the problem in the first place. And yes, you can achieve 100 percent recovery! You can get your life, your body, your natural beauty, your womanliness, and your sex life back! And yes, you can have babies!

Once you identify the cause or set of causes that conspired to upend your system, you can restore balance in your hormones and turn things around permanently. This book will help you do just that.

Learn from my success story

I have put together this guide to share my experiences, failures, learning, and successes. I would like to open your eyes to the diversity of polycystic ovarian syndrome as well as teaching you about all the natural interventions available for overcoming it. Here's my story.

I am 30 and on a journey to heal from polycystic ovarian syndrome. I used to be a professional dancer in ballet, tap and jazz. I have a university degree and am a passionate entrepreneur.

Although I was eating a healthy diet and taking supplements every day, I did not feel healthy. In fact, I was depressed. For eight long years my "normal life" consisted of terrible acne breakouts lasting 3 months, terrible menstrual pains and heavy bleeding. My weight was always fluctuating, I had zero sex drive, and I was moody. On top of all this, I have an underactive thyroid—only half of my thyroid gland works.

Then some really weird things started happening. I became so lethargic I did not want to get out of bed. Although my diet did not change, I started gaining weight. Massive, painful pimples appeared on my chin and jaw line. Then spread all over my face.

Thinking it was caused by hormone deficiency, I went on the birth control pill. But the acne persisted.

I visited my doctor and arranged for blood tests on all my hormones. The results came back and I was shocked. My estrogen, progesterone, estradiol levels—all vital female hormones—were so low they were out of normal range. The birth control pill was doing nothing.

What was going on? My doctor had no idea. She just suggested oral antibiotics for my skin.

The antibiotics didn't work. I decided to take my friend's advice and see an Endocrinologist—a doctor who specializes in women's hormones. After only one consultation, the Endocrinologist said my symptoms were screaming out that I had polycystic ovarian syndrome.

I had heard about this syndrome, since one of my cousins had it and was unable to fall pregnant with a second child.

As soon as I arrived home I tackled every resource I could find. I read about women who had overcome the symptoms, including facial acne, naturally. I learned about a regime that included eating healthy foods with low sugar content, avoiding toxic foods, taking certain supplements, and doing physical exercises. After only a month, my periods started to be regular for the first time since I was 16. I was getting the nutrients my body needed, and I started to feel better.

My Endocrinologist arranged a myriad of blood tests. She wanted to know the levels of every single hormone, and wanted to see if I was celiac or resistant to insulin. She also arranged scans on my ovaries and thyroid. In short, she wanted to know if I was suffering from polycystic ovarian syndrome as she thought.

On the day I came in to see my test results the Endocrinologist told me I had a small clump of small cysts in my right ovary. My hormone levels were all out of whack, and my thyroid levels were extremely low. It turned out she was right. She diagnosed me with polycystic ovarian syndrome and insulin resistance. She proceeded to write a prescription for regulating my insulin levels and then sent me away.

I had been waiting four weeks to see her. All I got was a fifteen minute debriefing. She did not take time to discuss how I was going to cope with all my symptoms. Was there a cure? Was there a support group? I needed comfort and support and all she gave me was a prescription that was going to address only one small aspect of my illness.

The drug she prescribed is called Metformin, and it is supposed to regulate blood sugar levels. Some women take it and they are fine. But after only two days I became terribly sick and lethargic. I craved sugar and was reaching for anything sweet in sight. One afternoon at the local mall, my blood sugar levels were so low I felt like I was going to pass out. I bought a salmon wrap and threw up within the hour. As I discovered, Metformin does not agree with sugar or high carb meals.

After continuing for another two days with horrible side effects, I decided to ditch Metformin and manage my insulin resistance without drugs. So many women who have tried Metformin know that it can be a horrible experience, making you lose weight unnaturally and causing low blood sugar levels.

Since then, I have regulated my insulin levels with diet and exercise. With normal insulin levels, my hormones are readjusting themselves and I am healing myself of PCOS.

Update over the past three years since this book was written:

My PCOS journey has been an interesting one. I have found more and more women I met are suffering with this dis-ease. It breaks my heart every time I meet someone with the same story as described above and say there is no hope, when indeed there is.

The simple fact is PCOS is caused by an imbalance of hormones and there is a root cause to all your issues that you need to dig deep to find out. Then it's as easy as having to learn how to manage this "issue" over your life otherwise the nasty side effects of PCOS will reappear.

At the end of the day PCOS is a lifestyle disease, your bad habits, poor food choices, stress, lack of exercise and self-love (which is not your fault) has lead you to this point. We only know as much as we know at the time, however the good news is that you can fix it!

I wrote this book for you to walk away with my many years of knowledge healing myself and at the point where now my body is able to bear children... naturally. I now live a life on my terms, not dictated by the horrible symptoms I had. Plus I am happy to report I am not hiding in my old house with a face full of acne anymore. I am in a loving relationship with my partner living in Perth Australia. I have an abundance of energy.

The past three years allowed me to discover I had adrenal fatigue issues, gene problems, gilberts disease of the liver (affecting the detoxification of toxins in my body), extremely sensitive insulin resistance issues, thyroid imbalances and more, which resulted in me ending up with cysts on my ovaries (PCOS) and infertility. All these "issues" are managed on day to day and guess what? I am as healthy as ever. I love my body, care for it and look after it every day to live a healthy, happy and abundant life and you will too.

I have discovered on my journey that food, air, good quality water and reducing stress are the most powerful ways to heal yourself. I'm feeling more alive and I know you will too, if you follow the simple steps in this book.

LISA'S STORY

At 33 years old, Lisa was diagnosed with PCOS. She had gained 10 kilos in six months, had cystic acne, chest hair and irregular periods. "Having fertility problems at such a young age was scary," says Lisa. "I thought I'd never be able to have a baby."

The doctors prescribed many medications including birth control. She proved allergic to everything. When they told her the disease was incurable, she became very depressed.

Lucky for her, Lisa researched all natural measures on how to heal PCOS naturally, and found the book *Heal My PCOS*. Having no other option, she contacted Melissa, and she was educated on the subject. "Melissa told me that everything we put in our bodies affects whatever we get out. Toxic foods cause diseases. She said it would not be easy but I would have to detoxify my body." Melissa put Lisa on a strict organic diet with a whole new approach to food. She bought a juicer and every three hours for three weeks she drank a combination of five carrots, one beet, one cucumber, two stalks of celery and one apple.

"It was the hardest thing I ever had to do," says Lisa, "but I did not complain once because I believed in it." The juice provided her with all the nutrients she needed while giving her digestive system a break after working so hard all these years. It allowed Lisa's body to purge all the toxins and help nurture her cells.

"The first three days were the hardest," says Lisa, "because my body was going through withdrawals from all the junk food I was eating. After that, it wasn't so bad! I got used to it!"

After three weeks, Lisa continued using the juicer but added different ingredients. She would make a nice fruit juice in the morning and vegetable juices for the rest of the day. The only 'food' she ate was organic vegetables for lunch.

And presto! "By Week 5, I got my menstrual cycle back! After that, it returned every 28 days, and all my other nasty symptoms disappeared. I lost 8 kilos!"

HEAL MY PCOS

She felt great. When she arranged for an ultrasound, the doctor said Lisa's ovaries were perfectly normal. "She could find NO signs of cysts anywhere!" Lisa said, "She was amazed and didn't know what to say. She had no explanation for how this could have happened! But I sure did!"

- 7 -

What is PCOS?

A health professional will diagnose the rather clunky term *polycystic ovarian syndrome* when you are not menstruating or your periods are irregular, when blood tests show abnormally high levels of androgens, and when an ultrasound shows cysts on the lining of your ovaries. Both the menstrual problems and the cysts are actually caused by the hormonal imbalance.

Put simply, PCOS is a hormone syndrome however it is also a metabolic condition. I refer to PCOS sometimes as "diabetes of the endocrine system".

Hormones are chemical messengers that control the way our body works. PCOS is a very common condition with up to 1 to 5 women of child bearing age being affected.

In medicine, a syndrome is a set of symptoms. But the other definition applies too: it's a set of behaviors. PCOS is one of the inevitable outcomes of Western culture — the way we eat, live and solve our problems. It's like our bodies' way of yelling at us, "Stop! This is just not going to work!"

What causes it?

Every illness is caused by an imbalance. Normally, two hormones, insulin and male type hormones are produced in higher levels, which results in problems such as periods becoming less regular (more or less often), hair growth on the face, acne, problems falling pregnant and more. I will discuss this more in the symptoms section of this book.

A woman may come down with PCOS when her personal choices and lifestyle are completely out of whack with her body's needs. Especially when it comes to diet. You may be eating a typical Western diet of processed foods and sugary snacks, sleeping poorly, suffering from constant stress, starving yourself to look thin, or experiencing wild ups and downs in your body weight.

These choices are actually considered normal in our society. But the prevalence of PCOS proves they are not healthy and they have serious consequences. They throw your whole system into chaos. For women, polycystic ovarian syndrome may be the result and it was in my case.

Types of PCOS

One of the main reasons I have written this book is that I believe there is a wide variety in the seven hormonal and metabolic influences and problems related to PCOS.

Each woman is an individual, and she needs to be viewed and treated as an individual. <u>No woman's PCOS is exactly the same as another woman's</u>.

I have broken down PCOS into three general types: Type 1, Type 2 and Type 3. These are categories that I have personally discerned to exist in the PCOS population, and ones that I have personally decided to use in my treatment and discussion of PCOS.

1.   Type 1 PCOS: insulin resistant

Usually found in an overweight woman, however can also occur in thinner women. This type is the focus of the medical community and comprises between 60% and 75% of the total PCOS population.

Indicators of Type 1:

- Being overweight, specifically in the abdomen
- Difficulty losing weight
- Acne
- Male pattern hair growth
- Hair growth on the face, thicker growth on arms, legs, abdomen and back.
- Male pattern hair loss
- Hair loss on the top of the head, hair thinning
- Irregular menstruation
- Blood markers:
  - High testosterone levels
  - Luteinising Hormone (LH): Follicle-stimulating Hormone (FSH) ratio higher than 1:1
  - Poor insulin sensitivity, glucose tolerance, and/or high fasting glucose

(Note: The majority of the book will revolve around this PCOS type as it is the leading cause of PCOS for women around the world, and was the type of PCOS I had).

Type 1 PCOS TAKE AWAY

Women with type I PCOS produce too much insulin as a result of eating the damaging foods characteristic of the standard Western diet. Excess insulin levels lead to excess testosterone production in the ovaries. These women are usually, though not always, overweight.

---

2. Type 2 PCOS: metabolically and/or psychologically stressed patients

Approximately 25% of the population suffer from this.

Indicators of Type B:

- Drastic weight loss (> ~10 kilos)
- Weight loss below level of body fat during puberty
- Daily exercise
- Obsession with exercise and/or body image
- Low body fat
- Extreme stress
- Poor sleep
- Blood markers:
  - Low Luteinizing Hormone (LH)
  - Low Follicle-stimulating Hormone (FSH)
  - Low Estrogen
  - Possibly high cortisol
  - Possibly high dehydroepiandrosterone sulphate (DHEA-S)

- ○ Higher than average testosterone
- ○ Low prolactin

Type 2 PCOS TAKE AWAY

Decreased body fat levels result in decreased estrogen and leptin levels, both of which are physical stressors and tell the brain that the body is starving. When the body is starving, it does not conduct reproductive cycles.

Psychological stress is another factor that tells the brain it is not a good time to have babies. For these reasons, all activities that cause metabolic and psychological stress can cause type 2 PCOS. These activities include under-eating, fasting, restricting calories or carbohy-drates, over-exercising, under-sleeping and failing to engage in stress reducing activities.

---

3. Type 3 PCOS: Hypothyroid patients

In addition to classic PCOS symptoms, hypothyroid symptoms include:

- Fatigue
- Difficulty losing weight
- Cold hands and feet
- Hoarse voice
- Gut issues
- Blood markers:
  - ○ Low or high thyroid stimulating hormone (TSH)

- ○ High thyroxine (T4)
- ○ Low triiodothyronine (T3)
- ○ High reverse T3
- ○ Hashimoto's Thyroiditis antibodies

Type 3 PCOS TAKE AWAY

Hypothyroidism can be a sole cause of PCOS and it very often is in the case of Hashimoto's Thyroiditis. It can also make pre-existing PCOS worse. For women who test positive for Hashimoto's, it is crucial to repair gut health with the anti-inflammatory natural foods diet as I have prescribed. They may also wish to supplement with thyroid hormone, depending on how advanced the disease is. All women, however, would do well to maximise thyroid health, being sure to reduce stress, sleep well, eat an appropriate amount of good fats and protein, and never be overly restrictive with diet or lifestyle choices.

On the following page is the progression from cause to effect:

Eating Habits, Lifestyle and Behaviours

Typical Western diet/food allergies	Starvation diet/food allergies	Severe weight loss	Lots of sugar	Stressful lifestyle	Lack of sleep

Body's Responses

Spike in insulin levels	Inflammation (bloating and fat storage)	Dysfunctional thyriod	Autoimmune Disease	Spike in cortisol	Adrenal Fatigue	Leaky gut

Hormonal Responses (Hypothalamus)

Increase in male hormones
Decrease in female hormones

Final consequences

Polystic ovarian syndrome
Cysts on the ovaries
No periods
Male pattern hair growth and/or baldness
Body weight volatility
No libido
Facial and body acne
Lethargy or depression
infertility

What tests do you need to have?

There is no single test to diagnose PCOS. Along my PCOS journey medical doctors unfortunately only performed minimal tests to diagnose my hormonal imbalances and metabolic issues.

I recommend seeing a health professional, such as a highly qualified naturopath to do a myriad of hormone tests on you—including blood, saliva tests and an iridology test.

These three tests helped me get to the root cause(s) of my PCOS so I could start managing my hormone levels myself moving forward. In my case, some of the issues that caused my PCOS included *(deep breath because it's a long list)*... adrenal fatigue, hypothyroidism, insulin resistance, elevated bilirubin (decreased capacity to detoxify through certain liver pathways), high testosterone, low progesterone and zero estrogen levels. When I found these were the causes to the PCOS syndrome, it was no wonder I was tired all the time, wasn't ovulating, infertile, had yellow hands, gained weight and acne all over my face and body!

A good health professional will take the following tests to find out if you have PCOS or if something else is causing your nasty symptoms, these tests will include:

Medical history. Your health professional will ask about your menstrual periods, weight changes and other symptoms.

Physical exam. Your health professional will measure your blood pressure, body mass index (BMI) and waist size. He or she also will check the areas of increased hair growth. You should try to allow the natural hair to grow for a few days before the visit.

Vaginal ultrasound (sonogram). Your doctor may perform a test that uses sound waves to take pictures of the pelvic area. It might be used to examine your ovaries for cysts and check the endometrium (en-do-MEE-tree-uhm) (lining of the womb). This lining may become thicker if your periods are not regular.

Pelvic exam. Your health professional might want to check to see if your ovaries are enlarged or swollen by the increased number of small cysts.

Blood tests. It is recommended to get a thorough blood test done through a regular medical doctor or through a good naturopath and/or natural practitioner.

It is important to check the two types of hormones in your bloodstream: free hormones and the hormones which are bound to proteins in the blood. I have had many women reach out to me, saying their hormones were in the "normal range" from their tests, however were still suffering from nasty symptoms. There are two ways of measuring these hormones: testing to see the number of "free" hormones in the bloodstream, and testing to see the "total overall number".

While doctors technically have the ability to test the blood for the free, unbound hormones, <u>most of the time doctors will only measure the total hormones in the blood.</u>

The problem is, while our total hormone count might be within normal range, if you have a high number of unbound hormones, then you are more than likely to end up with problems.

For example, with my blood test results back in 2013, my testosterone levels were within the normal range, however further testing from a naturopath, showed I had an elevated level of "free testosterone" in my body. This caused my severe acne (see image below). That's why just testing the total number of hormones isn't always giving you a true indication. If your doctor isn't able to help you, then another option is something called a saliva hormone test. Please keep reading.

My acne journey in 2013... This was the beginning of my acne. It progressively got worse to the point where I had painful acne all over my face, neck and body and hid in my house! My initial doctor had said my "levels were normal", when you can clearly see they were not. I had an elevated level of high "free testosterone" in my body. So please ask your doctor for total and unbound blood tests.

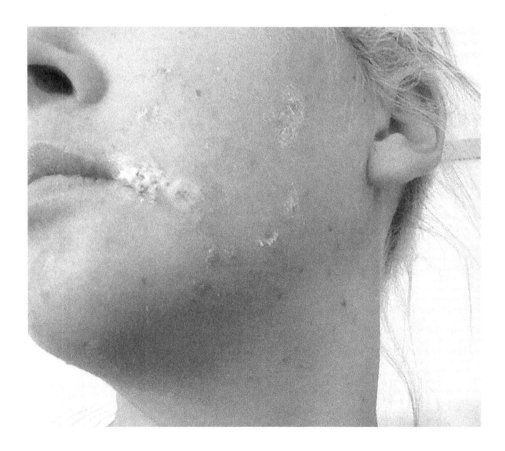

Most often, the following hormone levels are mea
considering a PCOS diagnosis. Ask your doctor
hormones!

- Lutenizing hormone (LH)
- Follicle-stimulating hormone (FSH)
- Total and Free Testosterone
- Dehydroepiandrosterone sulfate (DHEAS)
- Prolactin
- Androstenedione
- Progesterone
- Estrogen
- Thyroid stimulating hormone (TSH)
- Glucose
- Vitamin B12
- Iron

Salivary hormone test. Salivary hormone testing measures free, unbound hormones acting at a cellular level. Only the free hormones are able to easily diffuse into saliva and the body's tissues, so measuring the hormones in the saliva can give you an accurate picture of your hormone situation. I've been advised they are supposed to be more accurate in general for certain hormones, particularly estrogen.

Salivary hormone testing has been recognised by the World Health Organisation for over 30 years and is considered to be the most accurate method of identifying certain hormone levels. In my experience, the saliva test was the most profound test that I received to get a clear picture on what was happening.

he unfortunate thing about saliva hormone tests is they aren't cheap to get. However, they are more affordable than I once thought for the knowledge I had gained! A full hormone panel testing will cost around $200 AUD and this information will help you correct your hormone imbalances straight away. However, I recently discovered that you can have a full sex hormone panel testing done for half that, including a short consultation over the phone for interpretation, through an Australian based company called the Prana Health (currently only available if you call them).

Please contact me at info@healmypcos.com to receive a discount for your first consultation and it will include testing the following hormones:

- Cortisol
- DHEAs
- Testosterone
- Progesterone
- Oestrogens
- The three estrogens: estradiol, estrone, estriol
- Androstenedione
- DHT

Iridology test. Just like a meteorologist with weather, an Iridologist can detect when a storm is brewing with your health just by looking into your eyes. I highly recommend this alternative medicine technique as it detected that I had insulin resistance issues as well as issues with my ovaries. Iridology scientifically analyses patterns, colors, and other characteristics of the iris to determine information about your health and locates areas and stages of inflammation.

How to interpret your blood tests yourself

This is the one of the most exciting parts in the book! This will give you the power to determine your blood tests moving forward.

After you have received the results of your blood and saliva tests, you can now decode your results yourself! This knowledge will be worth its weight in gold moving forward in your life. You can refer back to this point in the book if you ever know your body is not right, because your hormones may get out of whack again... because you are only human!

This information has allowed me to keep a close check on my hormone levels for over three years now and happy and healthy along the way.

The ultimate guide to decoding your blood test results

Have you ever heard your doctor say... "Oh everything looks fine with your results" ... and you still feel like crap, have facial hair, have acne and no energy? It's what I heard and countless women hear from their doctors after receiving routine blood-test results.

And while you should listen to your doctor's analysis, you can also learn to decipher these mysterious blood tests yourself. It can yield surprising insights into your well-being and can help you spot—and work to fix—potential problems. This should be number one on every woman's get-healthy to-do list with being diagnosed with PCOS.

Blood test and normal ranges

Below I will converse what the normal ranges are for our hormones and how they work. This information has been confirmed by a highly qualified naturopath that has helped me heal along my journey.

Take a deep breath, grab your blood test results and compare the "normal ranges" to your own test results.

Do not freak out if yours is no-where near the normal ranges. At least you will then know where the imbalances are and you can then take the steps to reverse it and heal. Be kind to yourself...everything first starts with knowledge.

Here we go...

Lutenizing hormone (LH) and follicle stimulating hormone (FSH)

- **Normal range:** LH and FSH levels usually range between about 5-20 mlU/ml.

- Most women have about equal amounts of LH and FSH during the early part of their cycle. However, there is a LH surge in which the amount of LH increases to about 25-40 mlU/ml 24 hours before ovulation occurs. Once the egg is released by the ovary, the LH levels goes back down.

LH and FSH are the hormones that encourage ovulation. Both LH and FSH are secreted by the pituitary gland in the brain at the beginning of the cycle.

While many women with PCOS still have LH and FSH still within the 5-20 mlU/ml range, their LH level is often two or three times that of the FSH level. For example, it is typical for women with PCOS to have an LH level of about 18 mlU/ml and a FSH level of about 6 mlU/ml (notice that both levels fall within the normal range of 5-20 mlU/ml). This situation is called an elevated LH to FSH ratio or a ratio of 3:1. This change in the LH to FSH ratio is enough to disrupt ovulation. While this used to be considered an important aspect in diagnosing PCOS, it is now considered less useful in diagnosing PCOS, but is still helpful when looking at the overall picture.

Testosterone

- **Normal range:** The range for this is 6.0-86 ng/dl.
- All women have testosterone in their bodies.

There are two methods to measure testosterone levels:

- Total Testosterone
- Free Testosterone

Total testosterone refers to the total amount of all testosterone, including the free testosterone, in your body. The range for this is 6.0-86 ng/dl. Free testosterone refers to the amount of testosterone that is unbound and actually active in your body. This amount usually ranges from 0.7-3.6 pg/ml. Women with PCOS often have an increased level of both total testosterone and free testosterone. Furthermore, even a slight increase in testosterone in a woman's body can suppress normal menstruation and ovulation.

DHEA-S

- **Normal range:** It is normal for women to have DHEA-S levels anywhere between 35-430 ug/dl.

DHEA-S or dehydroepiandrosterone is another male hormone that is found in all women. DHEA-S is an androgen that is secreted by the adrenal gland. It is normal for women to have DHEA-S levels anywhere between 35-430 ug/dl. Most women with PCOS tend to have DHEA-S levels greater than 200 ug/dl.

Prolactin

- **Normal range:** Prolactin levels are usually normal in women with PCOS, generally less than 25 ng/ml.

Prolactin is a pituitary hormone that stimulates and sustains milk production in nursing mothers. Prolactin levels are usually normal in women with PCOS, generally less than 25 ng/ml. However, it is important to check for high prolactin levels in order to rule out other problems, such as a pituitary tumor, that might be causing PCOS-related symptoms. Some women with PCOS do have elevated prolactin levels, typically falling within the 25-40 ng/ml range.

Androstenedione (ANDRO)

- **Normal range:** ANDRO levels are between 0.7 - 3.1 ng/ml.

ANDRO is a hormone that is produced by the ovaries and adrenal glands. Sometimes high levels of this hormone can affect estrogen and testosterone levels.

Progesterone

- **Normal range:** If your Progesterone level is high (usually greater than 14 ng/ml) this means that ovulation did indeed occur and the egg was released from the ovary (check 7 days after ovulation).

Progesterone is produced by the corpus luteum after ovulation occurs. Progesterone helps to prepare the uterine lining for pregnancy. For women with PCOS, especially those who are trying to become pregnant using fertility medications, Progesterone levels are checked about 7 days after it is thought that ovulation occurred.

If the Progesterone level is high (usually greater than 14 ng/ml) this means that ovulation did indeed occur and the egg was released from the ovary. If the progesterone level is low the egg was probably not released. This test is especially important because sometimes women with PCOS can have some signs that ovulation is occurring however, when the progesterone test is done, it shows that ovulation did not occur. If this happens, your body may be producing a follicle and preparing you to ovulate, but for some reason the egg is not actually being released from the ovary. This information helps your physician possibly adjust fertility medication for the next cycle to encourage the release of the egg.

Estrogen

- **Normal range:** The range of normal varies widely depending on a person's age. For those between 20-29, the average is 149 pg/ml and will increase to 210 pg/ml for females 30-39. The level falls back to 152 pg/ml for women over 40 who are not yet in menopause. These levels are generalisations as the exact level varies on a daily basis and is closely tied to the various phases of the menstrual cycle.

Estrogen is the female hormone that is secreted mainly by the ovaries and in small quantities by the adrenal glands. The most active estrogen in the body is called estradiol. A sufficient amount of estrogen is needed to work with progesterone to promote menstruation. Most women with PCOS are surprised to find that their estrogen levels fall within the normal range (about 25-75 pg/ml). This may be due to the fact that the high levels of insulin and testosterone found in women with PCOS are sometimes converted to estrogen.

TSH

- **Normal range:** The normal TSH levels are (0.4-3.8 uIU/ml).

TSH stands for Thyroid Stimulating Hormone and is produced by the thyroid, a gland found in the neck. Women with PCOS usually have normal TSH levels (0.4-3.8 uIU/ml). TSH is checked to rule out other problems, such as an underactive or overactive thyroid, which often cause irregular or lack of periods and anovulation.

If you are being treated for a thyroid disorder, your TSH level will likely be kept between 0.5 and 4.0 mIU/L, except in these situations:

- For a pituitary disorder, a low TSH may be appropriate
- For thyroid cancer, a low TSH may be appropriate to prevent the thyroid cancer from coming back\
- The normal range for TSH is different for women who are pregnant. Your doctor may suggest that you take thyroid hormone, even if your TSH is in the normal range
- TSH values can vary during the day. It is best to have the test early in the morning.

Insulin and Glucose

Due to the recent research that PCOS is probably caused by insulin resistance, health professionals are beginning to check glucose levels as a factor when diagnosing PCOS. Most women with polycystic ovary syndrome should have a Fasting Plasma Glucose Test and a Glucose Tolerance Test at diagnosis and periodically thereafter. A high glucose level can indicate insulin resistance, a diabetes-related condition that contributes to PCOS.

Cholesterol

- **High cholesterol:** A high cholesterol level is considered greater than 200.

Researchers are also beginning to notice a connection between PCOS and heart disease; therefore, some physicians may want to look at your cholesterol levels when diagnosing and treating PCOS. Women with PCOS have a greater tendency to have high cholesterol, a major risk factor for developing heart disease. Cholesterol is a fat-like substance normally used by the body for form cell membranes and certain hormones. A high cholesterol level is considered greater than 200. Also, since the levels of good (high-density lipoproteins or HDL) and bad (low-density lipoproteins or LDL) are sometimes more indicative of a woman's risk for developing heart disease, these levels might also be assessed.

Too much bad cholesterol tends to increase the risk for plaque to build up in the arteries which can lead to a heart attack. Too much good cholesterol is believed to remove the cholesterol from building up in the arteries. Women with PCOS tend to have less good cholesterol and more bad cholesterol. In addition, triglyceride levels, another component of cholesterol, tend to be high in women with PCOS which further contributes to the risk of heart disease. Even if your health professional does not check your cholesterol levels when diagnosing PCOS, it is a good idea to have these levels checked periodically since women with PCOS have a greater chance of developing high cholesterol which can lead to heart disease.

I hope this guide on our hormone levels has helped you!

I know it started me off on the right foot to get my hormones in balance myself without checking in with a doctor all the time. Please refer back to it at anytime in the future as a guide, as I continually do to this day.

What are the symptoms?

Although the diagnosis normally requires the three factors — irregular periods, high levels of androgens and ovarian cysts to be present, the hormone imbalance can have additional symptoms that have serious impacts on a woman's life.

Symptoms can include:

- Infertility (inability to get pregnant) because ovulation is not occurring. PCOS is the most common cause of female infertility
- Infrequent, absent, and/or irregular menstrual periods
- Hirsutism (HER-suh-tiz-um) – increased hair growth on the face, chest, stomach, back, thumbs or toes
- Cysts on the ovaries
- Acne, oily skin or dandruff
- Weight gain or obesity, usually with extra weight around the waist
- Male-pattern baldness or thinning hair
- Patches of skin on the neck, arms, breasts or thighs that are thick and dark brown or black
- Skin tags – excess flaps of skin in the armpits or neck area
- Pelvic pain
- Adrenal fatigue
- Anxiety or depression
- Sleep apnea – when breathing stops for short periods of

time while asleep

Due to the hormonal imbalance and menstrual irregularity, you will not be ovulating and are therefore unable to get pregnant. However, you can once you know how to rebalance your hormones naturally. Being overweight is not always in itself a symptom. While most people diagnosed with the disease are overweight, some are of normal weight or are even underweight, which was my case – I was in the normal range for my age and height.

What causes PCOS?

Every illness is caused by an imbalance. As mentioned earlier, a woman may get PCOS when her personal choices and lifestyle are completely out of whack with her body's needs. This is the type of PCOS that is mainly recognised by the medical community. If you have PCOS and don't fit this regular mold and symptoms, you might have a hard time getting the right help you need, or even being diagnosed in the first place. There are three main kinds of PCOS, which I have talked about earlier, which all differ depending on the cause of your hormones getting out of whack and leading to the cysts, acne, facial hair and irregular cycles.

How did your system get out of balance?

The specific causes of your imbalance are unique. You may have a typical western diet comprised of empty calories. You may have consumed so much sugar over your lifetime that your body has lost its ability to process it. You may have a diet that is 80% flour and processed grains. You may have punished your body with excessive physical activity in the hopes of becoming "fit." You could be under immense stress at work. You could have chronic trouble sleeping peacefully through the night. You may have an underactive thyroid. You could even be exposed to too many xenoestrogens which are chemicals that are very similar to estrogens. Most of them are very strong and aggressive, beating the good estrogens to the receptors every time. What is scary is that they are in everything from your cosmetic makeup to your birth control to your water bottle.

'First consequences' of unhealthy choices

All of these factors trigger several responses in your body that I call 'first consequences'. Throughout this book, I will show how your behaviours and food choices cause these first consequences. All of them throw your hormones off balance and contribute to PCOS.

1.   High insulin levels

When your blood gets overloaded with sugar, it becomes toxic and threatens the overall balance of your blood and circulation. The sugar has to be put away somewhere so it does not interfere with normal functioning. So your pancreas distributes insulin, which acts as a vehicle to transport the sugar into your cells.

When this happens too often and with too much intensity—when there is too much sugar action and too much insulin action—the procedure starts to break down. The cells become less receptive to insulin and so the sugar lingers in the bloodstream along with the insulin.

Thus begins a chain reaction. With even more sugar stuck in the bloodstream, the pancreas manufactures and distributes more insulin, which tries again to deposit the sugar into the cells. Insulin begins to pile up in dangerous proportions and storage becomes more and more difficult.

The result is called insulin resistance, and often accompanies uncontrollable weight gain and acne. Even if a woman does not gain weight through this ordeal, her body suffers immense stress from the constant frustration of trying to store sugar and deal with high levels of insulin in the blood. Chronically high insulin levels can trigger chronically high testosterone levels.

I suffered with anorexia for many years. When I was 23 I weighed only 46 kilos. This is when I was first diagnosed with insulin resistance. I lived on a high-GI diet and in the end my body couldn't keep up, so I suffered with PCOS symptoms for the majority of my teenage life. Even if a woman doesn't gain weight, her body, like mine, will suffer immense stress from the constant frustration of trying to store sugar and deal with high levels of insulin in the blood.

Plus, when blood sugar swings are an everyday ongoing occurrence, eventually this leads to your cells being desensitized to insulin, which leads to even more insulin being released in order to get the glucose into the cells, and then even more androgens, and even more acne. This is why it's called "insulin resistance" and it is a big cause behind Polycystic Ovarian Syndrome and bad acne associated with androgen excess.

So to put it simply, a high sugar/high-GI diet will lead to a chronic overload of insulin, which means that testosterone levels are high, and under those circumstances ovulation is virtually impossible. I never had a proper period for many years due to this vicious cycle. Now I've learnt my lesson.

2. Inflammation (bloating)

Inflammation is what we often refer to as "fat." We seldom say "I'm eating too much junk food and I'm getting inflamed." But that's exactly what's happening in many cases, and that is why you can often lose so much weight so quickly by changing your diet. When you get a black eye, your skin tissue inflames in order to protect the wounded area. When you gain weight, it's often the same thing—your body is trying to protect itself from toxic invaders such as sugars, bad fats, certain vegetable oils and processed grains. You are storing substances that don't know where else to go, so they get lodged in your fat cells.

Inflammation puts a great deal of pressure on your metabolism. It spikes your insulin levels, interferes with normal thyroid function, and, in doing so, increases your production of testosterone.

3. Dysfunctional thyroid (hypothyroidism)

According to Dr Libby Weaver, one of Australasia's leading nutrition specialists, "the main function of the thyroid hormones is to convert the calories in food into useable energy for the body. If thyroid hormone levels drop below normal levels, metabolism inside cells slows down and energy levels drop. If thyroid hormone levels become too high, metabolism and all body processes speed up. These hormones also help control body temperature, heart rate and help regulate the production of proteins. A functioning thyroid gland is an essential component of having outstanding health and well-being.

In other words, your thyroid gland is absolutely essential to your hormonal balance, sexual energy, ovulation and fertility. It controls the metabolism, growth and development of each cell in the body. Its function is to deliver an energy-releasing hormone—called triiodothyronine (T3)—to your cells. When your blood lacks normal levels of T3, you have "hypothyroidism"—an underactive thyroid—and your reproductive system cannot work.

If you have an underactive thyroid, you will feel sluggish, fatigued and sleepy, yet sleep does not make you feel rested. You may feel increased sensitivity to cold, and may have dry skin, a puffy face and weak muscles.

The main cause of hypothyroidism is the typical Western diet. Other causes include mental and emotional stress, lack of sleep, restricted (starvation) diets, inflammation, and low carbohydrate diets.

An underactive thyroid means your reproductive system will not work properly or will not work at all. Hypothyroidism is one of the main precursors of PCOS.

In fact, says Dr. Weaver, hypothyroidism could almost be considered a "silent epidemic". Studies indicate that at least 10 percent—and possibly as many as 25 percent—of women over 60 will be affected with some degree of hypothyroidism.

4. Autoimmune disease

I've found more and more research that shows PCOS is often associated with Hashimoto's Thyroiditis or Hypothyroidism.

Hashimoto's disease is a common cause of hypothyroidism (underactive thyroid). It is an autoimmune condition. Immune system cells attack the thyroid gland, causing inflammation and, in most cases, eventual destruction of the gland. This reduces the thyroid's ability to make hormones. A recent study suggests that three to four out of every 10 PCOS women have impaired thyroid function, due to autoimmune thyroiditis (Hashimoto's Disease).

Consult your doctor for these tests to check if you have autoimmune issues:

1. Hormone test. Blood tests can determine the amount of hormones produced by your thyroid and pituitary glands. If your thyroid is underactive, the level of thyroid hormone is low.

2. An antibody test. Because Hashimoto's disease is an autoimmune disorder, the cause involves production of abnormal antibodies. A simple blood test may confirm the presence of antibodies against thyroid peroxidase (an enzyme important in the production of thyroid hormones).

5. Spikes in cortisol

When you are feeling worried or afraid or stressed, your brain halts the activity of your pituitary gland, whose job it is to distribute hormones to your blood. In the meantime, your adrenal glands kick into high gear, producing cortisol. Also called the stress hormone, cortisol spikes blood sugar. The adrenals also produce DHEA-S, another male hormone useful in scary circumstances.

This works well when you see a bear in the woods and you don't know what to do. But when you feel chronic stress and worry, the result is chronic hormone imbalance.

6. Adrenal Fatigue

Adrenal fatigue is purportedly when you've been so stressed out for such a long time that your adrenal glands become compromised and the output of stress hormones drops. This makes it extremely hard to deal with day-to-day stressors. This was a cause of my PCOS. I had such severe adrenal fatigue that I was falling asleep during the day and did not sleep well.

The problem with adrenal fatigue is it is a very controversial topic. It is not actually recognised as a real disorder by the medical community, who will treat the collective adrenal fatigue symptoms as if they are caused by something else, or say that they are "just stress".

If you've been stressed out for a long time, suspect you've got lower than normal adrenal output, or you have seen on your testing that your DHEA and cortisol levels are rock bottom, then the treatment is again pretty much the same as treating Type II PCOS and non-Hashimotos thyroiditis. The reason why I mention adrenal fatigue as a symptom of PCOS, because it wrecks havoic on your insulin resistance response and this is one of the leading underlying causes of PCOS.

On the following page is a table that shows how lifestyle and food choices throw your hormones out of whack. You may not notice symptoms for years.

Behaviour	First Consequences	Second Consequences
Eat a typical Western diet full of processed foods and empty calories and or food allergens	Your body does not get the nutrients it needs so you eat far bigger quantities. Your digestive organs may develop 'leaks' or holes.	Without essential nutrients, your basic hormones fall out of balance. Toxins sneak through the leaks and into your bloodstream instead of being processed and eliminated through the bowels.
Eat too many sugary foods	To deal with the sugar overload, your body produces extra insulin. Your insulin system may backfire. Your digestive organs may develop 'leaks' or holes.	Increased insulin levels cause your male hormone levels to shoot upwards. Toxins sneak through the leaks and into your bloodstream instead of being processed and eliminated through the bowels.
Eat too many baked goods, too much flour and processed grains	These empty calories deliver virtually no nutrition to your hungry cells. Your digestive organs may develop 'leaks' or holes.	Weight gain Toxins sneak through the leaks and into your bloodstream instead of being processed and eliminated through the bowels.

Behaviour	First Consequences	Second Consequences
Starve yourself or go on calorie-restricted diet	When you are constantly hungry, many of your body functions shut down in an effort to preserve body fat and essential nutrients rather than processing them for energy and reproduction.	No menstruation No body fat No sex drive Infertility
Exercise excessively	Your body interprets healthy estrogen levels as a signal that you have enough energy stored for fundamental functions. Too much exercise and weight loss causes estrogen to drop below a functioning level.	No menstruation

Behaviour	First Consequences	Second Consequences
Worry and stress constantly	Your adrenals go into high gear and you produce cortisol (called the stress hormone) in dangerous quantities. This spikes your blood sugar and your insulin levels. Higher cortisol also interferes with thyroid function. Stress also debilitates your pituitary gland, which regulates the female hormone functions.	Higher insulin levels lead to production of testosterone and other male hormones in the ovaries. Compromised pituitary function decreases the levels of estrogen, progesterone, and other female hormones. Decreased thyroid function leads to hormone imbalance.
Poor sleeping habits	When you sleep, your body repairs and rebalances itself. It affects thyroid function, among other things.	Lowered thyroid function leads to interruptions in hormone balance.

What do hormones have to do with cysts?

This is a very good question. There are two types of cysts that show up on women's bodies when hormones are off balance: facial or body acne, and ovarian cysts. Both are caused by abnormally high levels of male hormones but for different reasons.

When your female body is producing abnormal levels of androgen in proportion to your production of estrogen, your skin cells respond by producing more oil. The excess oil builds up and forms sacs on your skin that pressurize and become tender and painful. Women who have had clear skin all their lives can experience acne after menopause because their estrogen levels drop suddenly.

Cysts inside your ovaries, however, are not caused by a production of oil. They start out as healthy follicles in which your eggs develop. During normal ovulation, the egg is released from the follicle and is fertilized during sex or released via menstruation. When male hormones are high and female hormones are low, the normal cycles are not getting clear signals. The follicle won't open, the egg is not released, and the fluid is trapped in the follicle. It becomes a cyst.

What do hormones have to do with weight?

If you are too skinny for your frame, it can be a cause for hormonal imbalance. If you are too large for your frame, it can be both a cause and a result of hormonal imbalance. The key here is balance. Every human frame has its preferred balance of hormones, fat and muscle. If your weight is not normal for your frame, hormones will start to act up, and they get worse over time.

What are the chances of recovery?

You can FULLY recover from PCOS and restore hormonal balance if you change your diet and lifestyle. Other women have done it, and so can you! Read on!

AMBER'S STORY

Amber, the founder of overcomePCOS.com, was suffering from extreme hormone imbalance when she was just 18 years old. After months of excruciating pain, non-existent periods and unexplained weight gain, her doctor came in with the 'good news' that she had polycystic ovarian syndrome.

Within a year of the surgery, she ballooned up to 120 kilos, from size 10 to size 20. Her face was a constant mess of acne, and she was sprouting hair on her chin, neck, back and even breasts. In addition, she had horrible migraines and felt chronically tired no matter how much sleep she got.

Some of us have to hit rock bottom before we discover the path to our own redemption. For Amber, this was her rock bottom. She was miserable, and the depression was becoming unbearable. At this point, she knew that something had to change.

Several years later, after research, trial and error, Amber found the cure: eating a great diet and exercising. She changed her lifestyle and healed herself. Now 40 kilos lighter and wearing a size 8, Amber feels happier than she has in her entire life. Her skin is clear, she doesn't have the patches of hair anymore, and she has "plenty of energy to chase my children around the park!"

Your Guide for Healing

"PCOS is complicated. But healing is not. In healing type 1, type 2 and type 3 PCOS, what I did and each of you need to do is to de-stress, eat whole foods, adopt an insulin-sensitising, hormone-free diet, focus on nourishment and positivity, and achieve a healthy weight – Melissa"

1. Make yourself number one

It takes focus and dedication to heal yourself. You cannot rebalance your hormones if your career is Number One, your spouse or boyfriend is Number One, your education is Number One, your friends are Number One, or your kids are Number One.

If you care for other people more than you do for yourself, chances are you will not have the energy to heal yourself. Making yourself Number One is the only way to ensure long-term success in your relationships and career. You cannot be much help to your kids, spouse, employer, clients, friends or community if you are not looking after yourself first.

Take charge of your own healing

Forget about relying on someone or something else—your doctor, a health professional, a friend, a spouse, or a pill—to do it for you. They do not have any power to heal you. The power lies within you. We have to stop being patients and start being people.

We are taught to believe there is a magic solution for every medical problem, and the pharmaceutical industry likes to perpetuate this myth. It takes the power out of your hands and prompts you to reach for your wallet. It trains you to see the symptoms and ignore the causes, and this in turn tends to perpetuate the disease itself, which benefits big pharma, not you.

There may be others in your life who like to coddle you and solve your problems. It may give them a sense of control, and it gives you a feeling of being looked after. Whether the person is a spouse, a friend, a sibling or a parent, this co-dependence won't work when it comes time to heal.

When someone else is telling you what to do, you lose the inner clarity to zero in on exactly what you need, and you start doing things to satisfy their egos rather than doing what is right for you. Thank them for their caring, ask for their support, and tell them you are now going to take charge.

Get support

On the other hand, now is the time to ask for support. Start with those who are close to you: your spouse or partner, a close friend, a trusted co-worker, and members of your family whom you can trust. Be direct. Tell them your situation and the challenges ahead of you. Ask them to join you to provide moral support on your journey.

Do not approach anyone whom you do not trust. Do not approach anyone who tends to be negative or disparaging or critical. Focus only on those in whose company you feel affirmed, safe and happy: the people who appreciate you for who you are.

Your own children can be an immense source of support. Be open with them and they will rally around you.

There is no need to apologize or beg. You have nothing to apologize for. You are simply asking a favor. If you were in their position would you help? Of course you would. With very few exceptions, people want to help out in whatever way they can.

After all, you are only asking for support—someone you can talk to candidly. They don't need to do anything at all except be there for you.

COMMUNITY SUPPORT:

Please visit our loving community page:

www.facebook.com/healmypcos.

Here you can connect with like-minded ladies and my-self to help you through your PCOS healing journey.

Seek out alternative health professionals

Next, find one dedicated health professional who can support you in your journey. She could be a homeopath, naturopath, psychotherapist or life coach. Research the professionals in your area and see if you can get references. You want someone who is experienced, and eager to study your unique needs and the issues around hormonal imbalances. You need to feel comfortable in her presence, and feel that she is fully devoted to accompanying you on your journey.

It's tough to heal yourself when everyone around you is poisoning themselves from the typical Western diet of processed "foods", sugary snacks, beer and fast food. While you are transitioning your lifestyle, it's a good idea to decline some invitations and embrace others. Your true friends will understand. Everyone else will get the message and eventually adjust. In some cases, you will encourage people to follow your lead. Make yourself Number One and heal yourself, and your circle of friends will look after itself.

Be patient and gentle with yourself

Healing is a journey. There is no right and wrong, and there is no destination. It's all about loving yourself and nurturing yourself. The results will take care of themselves.

Our eating habits, addictions, expectations and cravings are not choices we made on our own. They are encouraged by virtually every respected sector of society. A cardiologist might consider a bottle of brandy a tasteful birthday gift. Your yoga instructor could offer muffins and coffee for a grand opening. Schoolteachers parrot the benefits of milk and cereal for breakfast. It takes resolve to run against this relentless current.

So be gentle with yourself, and remember you are the Captain and you answer to nobody else but you.

ALLY'S STORY - I got pregnant!

Ally was diagnosed with PCOS when she was only 15. Though her acne was embarrassing and she frequently missed periods, she did not bother about it until her maternal instincts came calling. She began to fear she could never have babies.

When she moved in with her new boyfriend, she decided it was time to heal herself. She drank lots of water, stopped drinking sodas, and stuck to a strict diet. She lost over 15 kilos. She attended fertility clinics and tried getting pregnant. She actually had a laparoscopy to remove her ovarian cysts. But after two years, she and her boyfriend had given up hope. They started to discuss artificial insemination, in vitro fertilization, and even surrogacy.

It was heart breaking for both of them. They desperately wanted kids. She blamed herself and got jealous when everyone else around her seemed to get pregnant at the drop of a hat.

And then she got pregnant.

"I was dumbstruck but my boyfriend Eddy didn't believe it. He told me to get an official test so we marched off to the pharmacy to buy one of those Clear Blue tests. I couldn't bring myself to look at it. Suddenly Eddy starts screaming. I burst into tears."

"Just yesterday," Ally continues, "I felt my baby move. What a miracle! I just want to encourage all my sisters. If it happened to me, it can happen to you. Keep healing yourself, and keep believing. You can be a Mother someday."

2. Nourish yourself

Once you have appointed yourself Captain of your healing, the primary way to turn your life around is to nourish your body with real food. Although there can be secondary causes of hormonal imbalance, garbage food is the main culprit. And while there are several other factors that will help you heal, real food is your most powerful medicine.

Eat real food

Your body loves real food. When you digest natural nutrients that your body can actually use, you feel satisfied, comfortable, and energized.

Real foods contain digestive enzymes that help you digest the food itself. The more organic or raw they are, the more digestive enzymes they contain. Processed foods contain virtually no digestive enzymes.

If you eat a tomato, you are giving yourself maximum goodness. When you eat tomato sauce cooked on top of pizza or spaghetti, you are not getting much tomato goodness.

When you switch to real food, you will notice wonderful new sensations. Your body feels much more energy after eating an apple than it does from eating a donut.

Invest more of your money in good food

Our typical Western diet fits perfectly with the typical Western lifestyle of rushing around and consuming everything in sight. Unlike other societies, eating in this part of the world is considered a consumer activity. It is based on the model that a bigger plate equals better value. At the same time, eating is often a bothersome afterthought: it's something we consider an interruption to other more important activities, such as work.

The economics of the Western food supply results in food that costs less and less per volume. A hundred years ago in North America, a typical family's food bill came to about 16% of their expenses. Today it is closer to 8%.

The implication is clear: Western society puts a very low value on food and eating. Ironically, obesity is rampant, as are hormonal imbalances.

To buck this trend, look at food as your most important expense. It's more important than your home, your job, your clothing and your transportation. To nourish yourself, you can expect to spend up to 20% of your monthly budget on food. There's no better place for your money.

Pursue variety

The variety in real food is virtually limitless. When you eat a meal with a variety of foods, you will not feel hungry again for several hours and your energy levels will remain relatively constant. When you try new foods, you give your body the kind of variety it craves rather than the same old stuff. You enable your body to find balance.

Eat right for your blood type

Eating right for my blood type changed my life. Only two months after adopting this new lifestyle, I had never felt better. Different diets work for different people, but if you haven't found one that works for you yet, this one might just be it.

I discovered this vital theory over the past few years on my healing journey. I can safely say that I was definitely not eating right for my blood type back in 2013 when I adopted a vegan lifestyle for the majority of that year, and in September my body shut down. I wasn't getting the necessary nutrients or fuel needed. It might have explained why I had always had trouble losing weight, had terrible skin and felt flat.

Food fads come and go, but the facts are clear: *everyone does not have the same basic nutritional needs*. We all know someone who is a strict vegetarian and thrives on that diet, while others swear by Atkins or similar low-carb plans. I've found and tested myself that your nutritional needs can be determined by your blood type.

When we discuss 'diet' in this book we are not necessarily talking about a weight loss plan, although weight loss may be a side benefit. We are actually discussing diet in the more traditional sense, meaning a way to eat.

My advice is to give this *way of life* a month and see if it makes a difference to you, especially if you are feeling lethargic and are having trouble falling pregnant. Get a blood test from your GP or ask your parents to find out what Blood type you are. I cannot stress enough how important this section is.

My blood type is O Positive, meaning I need to be eating more protein and less complex carbs. What blood type group are you?

Many people wonder about the importance of blood type and diet and this is important in the PCOS research debate. This is perhaps the reason why the nutrients that are harmful for people of one blood group are beneficial to another. The author of the bestsellers "Eat Right for Your Type", Dr. Peter D'Adamo, thinks an O positive blood type diet that can help people with type O blood to live a healthy life.

Type O

Most suited to animal proteins and intense physical exercise like jogging. O's are better for avoiding or limiting dairy products and grains. O's tend to be susceptible to developing asthma, hay fever, other allergies and arthritis.

Type A

Most suited to a vegetarian diet and fresh, organic foods. A's are best suited to calming exercise like yoga, and they are predisposed to heart disease, cancer, diabetes.

Type B

B's have a strong immune system, and tolerant digestive system, so they can eat most foods. They tend to resist many severe chronic degenerative illnesses, and are better suited to moderate physical exercise like cycling and swimming.

Type AB

Best suited to a combination of A and B. Type AB's tend to have the fewest problems with allergies, while heart disease, cancer, and anemia are medical risks for them.

It is important to note that gut bacteria composition is r to blood type. People of different blood types have different g bacteria; in fact certain bacteria are 50,000 times more likely to turn up in people with one blood type or the other. This originated from our ancestors whose digestive tracts developed to accommodate one type of diet over another. For example, the microbiome of certain people developed to break down carbohydrates much more efficiently (blood type A). People lacking this ability (blood type O) tend to store carbs as fat.

Gut health is so important and if your gut is not working properly then you need to possibly look at the foods you are eating and what is causing the irritation.

Blood type charts

Take a look at the food lists below; they are a guide for choosing the foods that will allow you to lose weight, reduce inflammation, increase energy and lead a longer, healthier life.

Type A

Type A's flourish on a vegetarian diet—if you are accustomed to eating meat, you will lose weight and have more energy once you eliminate the toxic foods from your diet. Many people find it difficult to move away from the typical meat and potato fare to soy proteins, grains and vegetables. But it is particularly important for sensitive Type A's to eat their foods in as natural a state as possible: pure, fresh and organic. I can't emphasize enough how this critical dietary adjustment can be to the sensitive immune system of Type A. With this diet you can supercharge your immune system and potentially short circuit the development of life threatening diseases.

Characteristics of Type A's - Best on Vegetarian Diet

	Comments	Most Beneficial	Food allowed	Food
Meats and Poultry	Type A's should eliminate all meats from their diet.		Chicken, cornish hens, turkey	Beef, veal, goose
Seafood		Carp, cod, grouper, mackerel, monkfish, pickerel, red snapper, rainbow trout, salmon, sardine, sea trout, silver perch, snail, whitefish, yellow perch	All kinds except those listed as not allowed	Anchovy, da, beluga, bluefish, bluegill bass, catfish, caviar, clam, conch, crab, crayfish, eel, flounder, frog, gray sole, haddock, hake, halibut, herring, lobster, lox, mussels, octopus, oysters, scallop, shad, shrimp, sole, squid, striped bass, tilefish, turtle
Dairy	Most dairy products are not digestible for Type A's		Yogurt, mozzarella, feta, goat cheese, goat milk, kefir, ricotta, string cheese	All other cheeses and milk

Characteristics of Type A's – Best on Vegetarian Diet				
	Comments	Most Beneficial	Food allowed	Food Not Allowed
Fats		Flaxseed oil, olive oil	Canola oil, cod liver oil	Oil of corn, cotton-seed, peanut, saf-flower and sesame
Nuts		Peanuts, pumpkin seeds	All kinds except those listed as not allowed	Brazil nuts, ca-shews, pistachios
Beans	These beans can cause a decrease in insulin pro-duction for Type A's.			Beans - copper, gar-banzo, kidney, lima, navy, red, tamarind
	Type As thrive on the vegetable proteins found in beans and legumes	Beans (aduke, azuki, black, green, pinto, red soy), lentils and black-eyed peas	All kinds except those listed as not allowed	
Grains	Type A's generally do well on cereals and grains. Se-lect the more concentrat-ed whole grains instead of instant and processed cereals.	Amaranth, buck-wheat		Cream of wheat, familia, farina, granola, grape nuts, wheat germ, seven grain, shredded wheat, wheat bran, durum wheat

Characteristics of Type A's - Best on Vegetarian Diet

	Comments	Most Beneficial	Food allowed	Food Not Allowed
Bread and Noodles	Type A's have a wonderful selection and choices in grains and pastas	Bread (essene, Ezekiel, soya flour, sprouted wheat), rice cakes, flour (oat, rice, rye), soba noodles, pasta (artichoke)	All kinds except those listed as not allowed	English muffins, bread (high-protein whole wheat, multi-grain), matzos, pumpernickel, wheat bran muffins, flour (white, whole wheat), pasta (semolina, spinach)
Vegetables	Type As are very sensitive to these vegetables. They have a strong deleterious effect on the Type A digestive tract. These vegetables enhance the immune system of Type A's	Garlic, onions, broccoli, carrots, collard greens, kale, pumpkin, spinach		Peppers, olives, potatoes, sweet potatoes, yams, all kinds of cabbage, tomatoes, lima beans, eggplant, mushroom

Characteristics of Type A's - Best on Vegetarian Diet

	Comments	Most Beneficial	Food allowed	Food Not Allowed
Vegeta-bles	Vegetables are vital to the Type A diet, providing minerals, enzymes and Antioxidants. Eat vegetables in as natural a state as possible (raw or steamed) to preserve their full benefits	Artichoke, chicory, greens (dandelion, swiss chard), horseradish, leek, romaine, okra, parsley, alfalfa sprouts, tempeh, tofu, turnip	All kinds except those listed as not allowed	
Fruits	Most fruits are allowed for Type A's, although try to emphasize more alkaline fruits can help to balance the grains that are acid forming in Type A's muscle tissues	Berries (blackberries, blueberries, boysenberries, cranberries), plums, prunes, figs	All kinds except those listed as not allowed	
	High mold counts of these fruits make it hard for Type A's to digest			Melons, cantaloupe, honeydew

MELISSA MADGWICK

Characteristics of Type A's - Best on Vegetarian Diet				
Fruits	Comments	Most Beneficial	Food allowed	Food Not Allowed
	Type A's don't do well on these fruits.			Mangoes, papaya, bananas, coconuts.
	These fruits are stomach irritant for Type A's, and they also interfere with the absorption of minerals.			Orange, rhubarb, tangerines.
	The digestive enzyme in this fruit is an excellent digestive aid for Type A's.	Pineapples, cherries, apricots.		
	These fruits exhibit alkaline tendencies after digestion which has a positive effects on the Type A stomach.	Grapefruit, Lemon.		

Characteristics of Type A's - Best on Vegetarian Diet	Comments	Most Beneficial	Food allowed	Food Not Allowed
Spices	The right combination of spices can be powerful immune-system boosters for Type A's.	Tamari, miso, soy-sauce, garlic, ginger.		
	Good source of iron, a mineral that is lacking in the Type A Diet.	Blackstrap molasses.		
	Avoid these because the acids tend to cause stomach lining irritation.			Vinegar, pepper (black, cayenne, white), capers, plain gelatin, wintergreen.
Condiments	These products should be avoided because Type A's have low levels of stomach acid.			Ketchup, mayonnaise, pickles, relish, worcestershire sauce.

Characteristics of Type A's - Best on Vegetarian Diet

	Comments	Most Beneficial	Food allowed	Food Not Allowed
Beverages	These beverages help to improve the immune systems for Type A's.	Hawthorn, aloe, alfalfa, burdock, echinacea, green tea, red wine (1 glass / day).		
	These beverages help Type As to increase their stomach-acid secretions.	Ginger, slippery elm, coffee (1 cup / day).		
	These don't suit the digestive system of Type A's, nor do they support the immune system.			Beer, distilled liquor, seltzer water, soda, black tea.

Type O

Type Os high stomach-acid content, can digest meat easily. They thrive on intense physical exercise and animal proteins. They do not do well with dairy and grain products. The leading factor in weight gain for Type Os is the gluten found in wheat germ and whole wheat products. Type O have a tendency to have low levels of thyroid hormone and unstable thyroid functions, which cause metabolic problems and weight gain. Some ancient grains are allowed such as spelt, Dr DaMo explains that spelt is a flowering grass. Its fruit is an ancient cereal grain and belongs to the same family of plants that include bamboo, rice, sugarcane and modern wheat. It is easily digestible and has slightly higher protein content than wheat. Often, it can be tolerated by those with wheat allergies.

Characteristics of Type O – Best on High Protein Diet

	Comments	Most Beneficial	Food allowed	Food Not Allowed
Protein	The more stressful your job or demanding your exercise program, the higher the grade of protein you should eat.	Beef, lamb, mutton, veal, venison.		
	Type O's can efficiently digest and metabolize meats.		Any meat except for those listed as not allowed.	Bacon, Ham, Goose, Pork.
	Cold-water fish are excellent for Type O's. Many seafoods are also excellent sources of iodine, which regulates the thyroid function.	Cod, herring, mackerel.	Any fish or seafood except for those listed as not allowed.	Barracuda, pickled herring, catfish, smoked salmon, caviar, octopus, conch.
Dairy	Type O's need to severely restrict the use of dairy products and eggs.		Butter, ghee, farmer, feta, mozzarella, goat cheese.	All other dairy products and yogurts.

Characteristics of Type O - Best on High Protein Diet				
	Comments	Most Beneficial	Food allowed	Food Not Allowed
Fat	Type O's respond well to oils.	Olive oil, flaxseed oil.	Canola oil, sesame oil.	Corn oil, peanut oil, cottonseed oil, safflower oil.
Nuts	These foods should in no way take the place of high-protein meats, and they are high in fat especially if you are over-weight.	Pumpkin seeds, walnuts.	All kinds except those listed as not allowed.	Brazil, cashew, peanut, pistachios, poppy seeds.
Beans	Type O's don't utilize beans particularly well. They tend to make muscle tissue slightly less acidic and inhibit the metabo-lism of other nutrients.	Aduke beans, Azuki beans, Pinto beans, Black-eyed peas.	All kinds except those listed as not allowed.	Beans - copper, kid-ney, navy, tamarine. Lentils - domestic, green, red.

Characteristics of Type O - Best on High Protein Diet

	Comments	Most Beneficial	Food allowed	Food Not Allowed
Grains	Type O's do not tolerate whole wheat products at all.	Essene bread, Ezekiel bread.	Amaranth, buckwheat, rice, kamut, kasha, millet, spelt.	Corn, gluten, graham, wheat (bulgur, durum, sprouted, white and whole, germ and bran) farina, oat, seven-grains, or any products such as flour, bread and noodles made with these grain products.
Vegetables	These vegetables inhibit the thyroid function for Type O's.			Brassica family: cabbage, Brussels sprouts, cauliflower, mustard greens.
	These vegetables help the blood clot. Type O's lack several clotting factors and need vitamin K to assist in the process.	Kale, collard greens, romaine lettuce, broccoli, spinach.		

Characteristics of Type O - Best on High Protein Diet

	Comments	Most Beneficial	Food allowed	Food Not Allowed
Vegeta-bles	These vegetables irritate the digestive tract and the high mold count can aggravate Type O hyper-sensitivity problems.			Alfalfa sprouts, shitake mushrooms, fermented olives.
	These vegetables can cause arthritic conditions in Type O's.			Nightshades: eggplant, potatoes.
	This vegetable affects the production of insulin, often leading to obesity and diabetes for the Type O's.			Corn.
	This fruit agglutinates all blood types but Type O's.		Tomatoes.	

Characteristics of Type O – Best on High Protein Diet

	Comments	Most Beneficial	Food allowed	Food Not Allowed
Vegetables		Artichoke, chicory, dandelion, garlic, horseradish, kale, leek, okra, onions, parsley, parsnips, red peppers, sweet potatoes, pumpkin, seaweed, turnips.	All kinds except those listed as not allowed.	Avocado.
Fruits	Dark red, blue and purple fruits tend to cause an alkaline reaction in the digestive tract, and therefore balance the high acidity of the Type O's digestive tract to reduce ulcers and irritations of the stomach lining.	Plums, prunes, figs.		

Characteristics of Type O - Best on High Protein Diet

	Comments	Most Beneficial	Food allowed	Food Not Allowed
Fruits	These fruits contain high mold counts which can aggravate Type O's hypersensitivity problems (allergies).			Melons, cantaloupe, honeydew.
	These fruits are high in acid content which may irritate the acidic stomach of Type O's.		Grapefruit, most berries.	Oranges, tangerines and strawberries, blackberries, rhubarb.
	Fruits are not only an important source of fiber, minerals and vitamins, but they can be an excellent alternative to bread and pasta for Type O's.		All kinds except those listed as not allowed.	

Characteristics of Type O - Best on High Protein Diet

	Comments	Most Beneficial	Food allowed	Food Not Allowed
Fruits	Type O's are extremely sensitive to this fruit.			Coconut and coconut-containing products.
Spices	Rich source of Iodine to regulate the thyroid gland.	Kelp-based seasonings, iodized salt.		
	Soothing to the digestive tracts of Type O's.	Parsley, curry, cayenne pepper.		
	Irritants to the Type O stomach.			White and black pepper, vinegar, capers, cinnamon, cornstarch, corn syrup, nutmeg, vanilla.
Condiments			Chocolate, honey, cocoa.	Ketchup, pickles, mayonnaise, relish.
Beverages		Seltzer water, club soda and tea.	Wine.	Beer, coffee, distilled liquor, black tea.

Type B

For Type B's the biggest factors in weight gain are corn, wheat, buckwheat, lentils, tomatoes, peanuts and sesame seeds. Each of these foods affect the efficiency of your metabolic process, resulting in fatigue, fluid retention, and hypoglycemia—a severe drop in blood sugar after eating a meal. When you eliminate these foods and begin eating a diet that is right for your type, you blood sugar levels should remain normal after meals. Another very common food that Type B's should avoid is chicken. Chicken contains a Blood Type B agglutinating lectin in its muscle tissue. Although chicken is a lean meat, the issue is the power of an agglutinating lectin to attack your bloodstream and potentially lead to strokes and immune disorders. Dr. D'Adamo, from his studies, suggests that you wean yourself off chicken and replace it with highly beneficial foods such as goat, lamb, mutton, rabbit and venison. Other foods that encourage weight loss are green vegetables, eggs, beneficial meats, and low fat dairy. When the toxic foods are avoided and replaced with beneficial foods, Blood Type B's are very successful in controlling their weight.

Characteristics of Type B's - Best on Balanced Omnivores Diet

	Comments	Most Beneficial	Food allowed	Food Not Allowed
Meat and Poultry	These meats contain a Type B blood agglutinating lectin.			Chicken, cornish hens, duck, goose, partridge, quail, pork..
	These meats help to boost the immune system.	Lamb, mutton, venison, rabbit.		
	Give up chicken, but use these meats instead.		Beef, pheasant, turkey, veal.	
Seafood	Deep-ocean fish and white fish are great for Type B's.	Cod, salmon, flounder, halibut, sole, trout.	All kinds except those listed as not allowed.	
	These seafood are poorly digested by Type B's. They are disruptive to the Type B system.			All shellfish (crab, shrimp, lobster, mussels, oysters, crayfish, clam, etc), anchovy, barracuda, beluga, eel, frog, lox, octopus, sea bass, snail, striped bass, turtle, yellowtail.

Characteristics of Type B's - Best on Balanced Omnivores Diet				
	Comments	**Most Beneficial**	**Food allowed**	**Food Not Allowed**
Dairy	Type B is the only blood type that can fully enjoy a variety of dairy foods. That's because the primary sugar in the Type B antigen is D-galactosamine, the very same sugar present in milk.	Cottage cheese, farmer, feta, goat cheese and milk, kefir, mozzarella, ricotta, milk, Yogurt.	All kinds except those listed as not allowed.	American cheese, Blue cheese, Ice cream, string cheese.
Fats	The oils not allowed contain lectins that are damaging to the Type B digestive tract.	Olive.		Canola, corn, cottonseed, peanut, safflower, sesame, sunflower.
Nuts	Most nuts and seeds are not advisable for Type Bs. They contain lectins that interfere with Type B insulin production.		All kinds except those listed as not allowed.	Cashews, filberts, pine, pistachio, peanuts, pumpkin seeds, sesame seeds, sunflower seeds.

Characteristics of Type B's - Best on Balanced Omnivores Diet				
	Comments	Most Beneficial	Food allowed	Food Not Allowed
Beans	These beans interfere with the production of insulin for Type B's.			Lentils, garbanzos, black-eyed peas, Beans (pintos, duke, azuki, black).
Grains	Wheat reduces insulin efficiency and failure to stimulate fat "burning" in Type B's.			Wheat (bran, germ bulgur, durum, whole and white), shredded wheat, cream of wheat or any products such as flour, bread and noodles made with these grain products.
	Rye contain a lectin that settles in the vascular system causing blood disorders and potentially strokes.			Rye and any products such as flour, bread and noodles made with these grain products.

Characteristics of Type B's - Best on Balanced Omnivores Diet				
	Comments	Most Beneficial	Food allowed	Food Not Allowed
Grains	These contribute to a sluggish metabolism, insulin irregularity, fluid retention and fatigue.			Buckwheat, corn (cornflakes, cornmeal) and any products such as flour, bread and noodles made with these grain products
		Millet, oatmeal (bran, flour), puffed rice, rice (bran, flour), spelt.	All kinds except those listed as not allowed.	Amaranth, barley, kasha, seven-grain, wild rice, couscous.
Bread		Bread (brown rice, essence, ezekiel, wasa), fin crisp, millet, rice cakes.	All kinds except those listed as not allowed.	Bagels, muffins (corn and bran), bread (multi-grain rye, whole wheat), soba noodles, wild rice, couscous.
Vegeta-bles	This vegetable contain lectins that irritate the stomach lining of Type B's.			Tomatoes

Characteristics of Type B's - Best on Balanced Omnivores Diet				
	Comments	Most Beneficial	Food allowed	Food Not Allowed
Vegeta-bles	This vegetable has insulin- and metabolism-upsetting lectins for Type B's.			Corn.
	The mold in this can trigger allergic reactions.			Olive.
	These vegetables contain magnesium, an important antiviral agent to help Type B's fight off viruses and autoimmune diseases.	Green leafy vegetables.	All kinds except those listed as not allowed.	Artichoke, avocado, corn, olives, pumpkin, radishes, sprouts, tempeh, tofu, tomato.
Fruits	Pineapple has enzymes that help Type B's to digest their food more easily.	Pineapples.		

Characteristics of Type B's - Best on Balanced Omnivores Diet				
	Comments	Most Beneficial	Food allowed	Food Not Allowed
Fruits	Avoid these fruits as they interfere with your digestive system.			Coconuts, persimmons, pomegranates, prickly pear, rhubarb, starfruit.
		Bananas, cranberries, grapes, papaya, plums.	All kinds except those listed as not allowed.	
Spices	Sweet herbs tend to be stomach irritants to the Type B's.			Barley malt sweeteners, corn syrup, cornstarch, cinnamon.
	Type B do best with warming herbs.	Ginger, horseradish, curry, cayenne pepper.	All kinds except those listed as not allowed.	
	Avoid these spices also.			Allspice, Almond extract, Gelatin, Pepper (black and white).

Characteristics of Type B's - Best on Balanced Omnivores Diet				
	Comments	Most Beneficial	Food allowed	Food Not Allowed
Condi-ments				Ketchup
Beverages	Generally Type B's don't reap overwhelming benefits from most herbal teas.	Ginger, peppermint, raspberry leaf, rose hips, sage, green teas.		Aloe, coltsfoot, corn silk, fenugreek, gentian, golden-seal, hops, linden, mullein, red clover, rhubarb, senna, shepherd's purse, skullcap.
	This is highly recom-mended for Type B's because it seems to have a positive effect on the nervous system.	Ginseng.		
	This has antiviral prop-erties.	Licorice.		Distilled liquor, Selt-zer water, Soda.

Type AB

Type AB reflects the mixed inheritance of their A and B genes. According to Dr. D'Adamo, "Type AB has Type A's low stomach acid, however, they also have Type B's adaptation to meats." Therefore, you lack enough stomach acid to metabolize meats efficiently and the meat you eat tends to get stored as fat. Because type AB has both the A and the B blood type antigens, foods that contain chemicals called lectins are more likely to react with the tissues and cells of type AB than any of the other blood types.

Characteristics of Type AB - Best on Mixed Diet in moderation

	Comments	Most Beneficial	Food allowed	Food Not Allowed
Meat and Poultry	Type AB do not produce enough stomach acid to effectively digest too much animal protein. So the key is portion size and frequency.	Lamb, mutton, rabbit, turkey.	All kinds except those listed as not allowed.	Beef, chicken, cornish hens, duck, goose, pork, partridge, veal, venison, quail.
	Cured meats can cause stomach cancer in Type AB's with low levels of stomach acid.			
Seafood	If you have family history of breast cancer, introduce snails (Helix pomatia) into your diet.	Tuna, cod, grouper, hake, mackerel, mahimahi, monkfish, ocean perch, pike, porgy, trout, red snapper, sailfish, pickerel, sardine, shad, snail, sturgeon.	All kinds except those listed as not allowed.	All shellfish (crab, shrimp, lobster, mussels, oysters, crayfish, clam, etc), anchovy, barracuda, beluga, bluegill bass, flounder, haddock, halibut, herring, eel, frog, lox, octopus, sea bass, striped bass, turtle, yellow-

Characteristics of Type AB - Best on Mixed Diet in moderation

	Comments	Most Beneficial	Food allowed	Food Not Allowed
Dairy	Cultured and soured products are easily digested for Type AB's.	Yogurt, kefir, non-fat sour cream, egg, mozzarella, goat cheese and milk, ricotta.	All kinds except those listed as not allowed.	American cheese, blue cheese, brie, buttermilk, camembert, ice cream, parmesan, provolone, sherbet, whole milk.
Fats	Use sparingly.	Olive.		Oil (corn, cotton-seed, safflower, sesame, sunflower).
Nuts	Powerful immune booster for Type A and Type AB.	Peanut, walnuts.		
	Type AB's tend to suffer from gallbladder problems, so nut butters are preferable to whole nuts. Also eat small amounts with caution.		All kinds except those listed as not allowed.	Filberts, poppy seeds, pumpkin seeds, sesame seeds, sunflower seeds.

Characteristics of Type AB - Best on Mixed Diet in moderation			
	Comments	Most Beneficial	Food allowed	Food Not Allowed
Beans	These beans are important cancer-fighting food for Type AB. They are known to contain cancer-fighting antioxidants.	Lentils.		
	These beans slow insulin production in Type AB.			Kidney beans, lima beans.
		Beans (navy, pinto, red, soy).	All kinds except those listed as not allowed.	Beans (aduke, azuki, black, fava, garbanzo) black-eyed peas.

Characteristics of Type AB - Best on Mixed Diet in moderation			
	Comments	Most Beneficial	Food allowed	Food Not Allowed
Grains	The inner kernel of the wheat grain is highly acid forming for Type AB. Wheat is not advised if Type AB is trying to lose weight. The inner kernel of wheat grain is alkaline in Type O's and B's, it becomes acidic in Type A's and AB's.	Millet, Oat bran, Oatmeal, Rice Bran, Puffed rice, Rye, Spelt and sprouted wheat and any products such as flour, bread and noodles made with these grain products.	All kinds except those listed as not allowed.	Buckwheat, corn (any products such as flour, bread and noodles made with these), kamut, kasha, soba noodles, artichoke pasta.
	Type AB benefits from a diet rich in rice rather than pasta.	All kinds of rice and any products such as flour, bread and noodles made with these.		

Characteristics of Type AB - Best on Mixed Diet in moderation				
	Comments	Most Beneficial	Food allowed	Food Not Allowed
Vegeta-bles	Fresh vegetables are an important source of phytochemicals which have a tonic effect in cancer and heart disease prevention, these diseases afflict Type AB more often as a result of weaker immune system.	Broccoli, beets, cauliflower, celery, green leafy vegs, cucumber, eggplant, garlic, maitake mushroom, parsley, parsnips, sweet potatoes, alfalfa sprouts, tempeh, tofu, all types of yams.	All kinds except those listed as not allowed.	Artichoke, avocado, all type of corns, lima beans, black olives, all kind of bell peppers, radishes, mung bean sprouts, radish sprouts.
Fruits	Emphasize the more alkaline fruits to balance the grains that are acid forming in Type AB muscle tissues.	All kinds of Grapes and Plums, Berries (cranberries, Gooseberries, Loganberries), Cherries.		

Characteristics of Type AB - Best on Mixed Diet in moderation

	Comments	Most Beneficial	Food allowed	Food Not Allowed
Fruits	Tropical fruits doesn't agree with Type AB. But pineapple is an excellent digestive aid for Type AB.	Pineapples.	Mangoes, Guava, Coconuts, Bananas.	
	Oranges are stomach irritants for Type AB, they also interfere with the absorption of important minerals. But Grapefruit exhibit alkaline tendencies after digestion. And lemons aid digestion and clearing mucus from the system.	.Grapefruits, Lemons		Oranges.
	Vitamin C-rich fruits help prevent stomach cancer because of the antioxidant properties of vitamin C.	Kiwi	All kinds except those listed as not allowed.	

Characteristics of Type AB - Best on Mixed Diet in moderation			
	Comments	Most Beneficial	Food allowed	Food Not Allowed
Spices	Sea salt and kelp should be used in place of salt. Kelp has immensely positive heart and immune system benefits.	Kelp, Miso, Curry.	All kinds except those listed as not allowed.	Allspice, almond extract, anise, barley malt, capers, corn-starch, corn syrup, gelatin, tapioca.
	The ingredients are acidic.			Vinegar, pepper (white, black, cayenne, red flakes).
	This is a potent tonic and natural antibiotic for Type AB.	Garlic, horseradish, parsley.		
Beverages	Type AB can employ these herbal teas to rev up the immune system.	Alfalfa, burdock, chamomile, echinacea, green tea.		

Characteristics of Type AB – Best on Mixed Diet in moderation				
	Comments	**Most Beneficial**	**Food allowed**	**Food Not Allowed**
Beverages	These herbal teas and beverages build protections against cardiovascular disease and cancer.	Hawthorn, licorice, red wine (1 glass/day).		
	These herbal teas aid in absorption of iron and prevent anemia.	Dandelion, burdock root, strawberry leaf.		
	Coffee increases stomach acid and has the same enzymes found in soy.	Coffee or decaf coffee (1 cup / day) and alternate day use green tea.		Distilled liquor, sodas, black tea.

Enjoy shopping for real food

Try new vegetables and organic meats. Don't go for volume: think instead of quality. Talk about the food you are going to eat. Learn where it comes from and how it is harvested.

Make your kitchen your sanctuary

Since eating and drinking is the most important human activity and the key to healing yourself, make your kitchen the center of your life. Serenade the space with music. Talk to your friends on the phone while dicing up veggies and marinating meat. Consider a new paint job, new curtains, a new countertop or sink, even new tea towels. Do whatever you need in order to feel comfortable as you enjoy your food at your own table.

Make each meal an experience

It's not just the actual food that your body loves. It also loves the activity of eating. Here in the Western world, we have forgotten this experience. The rest of the world seems to know it! Meals are the focal points of culture and socializing the world over.

Chewing, for instance, gives your brain the feeling of well-being. Bite into an apple or a piece of celery and see how it boosts your mood! Tastes that surprise your taste buds and glands are a delight for your whole body. By experiencing different textures and chemical combinations, you are giving your body a chance to wake itself up. In the act of processing the foods and transforming the nutrients to glucose, your body is doing what it has been trained to do for millennia. It does this very well. Your body is happy doing it.

You will notice that when you slow down, savor your meal, chew slowly and thoroughly, you naturally hydrate your body and you won't need any beverage to wash anything down. That's what your saliva is for. It's the first step in digestion and it performs a similar function to your stomach chemicals.

Drink lots of water

Water is a natural cleansing and healing agent all on its own. When your body is poorly hydrated, it cannot digest food properly, and the nutrients will not do their maximum work. A dry body also means your immune system is at risk.

Drinking water needs to be a daily habit. As soon as you wake up, drink 8 to 16 ounces of water—the equivalent of a water bottle. Don't use plastic bottles, however.

Don't drink water while you are eating or directly after a meal. Water interferes with the natural chemicals that your stomach uses to fully digest and process food. It will also give you gas.

Drink another full glass of water before you go to bed.

I encourage you to not to drink from plastic bottles. In third-party testing, bottled water showed traces of bacteria, chemicals, fluoride and endocrine disruptors such as BPA and PETE (or PET). That's a whole other story! Drink a full glass of water 30 minutes before your meals and in between meals to aid with digestion.

It takes some getting used to, but water will eventually replace all those drinks you have used to quench your thirst. It will replace soda and juices and milk, for sure. And you will notice a difference in your skin, your sinuses and your overall feeling of well being.

Eat balanced meals

Make sure each meal has a good portion of protein, carbohydrates and fats. For example, a good breakfast could be egg whites (protein), oatmeal (carbohydrate), and almonds (fats). A good lunch would be turkey (protein), arugula and tomato (carbohydrates) and coconut oil (fats). Each type of food helps the others digest properly.

Concentrate on foods with low sugar

"Sugar, remember, is one of the biggest causes of PCOS. However, it is not just sweet foods you need to be wary of. Many starchy foods which are not at all sweet are very easily broken down into sugar by the body. By choosing mainly foods that are neither sugary nor easily converted into sugars, you avoid spiking your blood glucose level, and this helps restore normal insulin levels.

This in turn helps you rebalance your hormones and get back to robust health.

You can help yourself by learning how much sugar natural foods contain, and by learning which carbohydrate foods have a marked effect on blood sugar levels. The technical term for sugar in foods and in your blood is glycaemia. A food that is slowly broken down by the body and does not cause a rapid rise in blood glucose levels is low on the "glycemic index," or GI. You want to stick with "low GI" foods and minimize your consumption of "high GI" foods. You can decrease the glycemic index of your whole meal or your whole diet by replacing high GI foods with low GI foods.

It does not mean you cannot eat foods with a high sugar content. It just means that you are going to see more progress if you avoid them or drastically reduce the amount you eat.

As the chart on the next page shows, there is no shortage of delicious favorite foods that are low on the glycemic index.

Here's more good news: low GI foods do more than keep your insulin in check. Since your digestive system processes these foods more slowly, you will feel full for hours, and feel more satisfied than you would with "sweeter" foods. This will help regulate both your diet and your energy levels.

On the next three pages is a chart of some typical foods and their rating on the glycemic index (the numbers below in the table correspond to proportionate units of glucose found in certain foods). Notice that I have not included any wheat-based or processed foods such as pastries, pasta, or boxed cereals. As Chapter 3 will show, those are foods you want to stay away from entirely.

Low glycaemic index (55 and under)

Make these foods your staples!

Fruits	Vegetables	Legumes + Grains	Other
cherries	peas	kidney beans	nuts
plums	carrots	butter beans	coconut milk
grapefruit	eggplant	chick peas	egg
peaches	broccoli	(hummus)	good fats
apples	cauliflower	navy beans	seafood
pears	cabbage	lentils	meat (2-3
dried apricots	mushrooms	pinto beans	times a week)
grapes	tomatoes	black eyed	
kiwi	lettuce	beans	
oranges	green beans	yellow split	
strawberries	sweet peppers	peas	
prunes	onions	brown/black	
avocado	sweet potatoes	rice	
coconut	yams	oats	

Medium glycaemic index (56 to 69)

Go easy on these foods.

Fruits	Vegetables	Legumes + Grains	Other
mango sultanas bananas raisins papaya figs pineapple	beets baked potatoes	wild rice white basmati rice	honey

High glycaemic index (70 and over)

Avoid these foods.

Fruits	Vegetables	Legumes + Grains	Other
watermelon dates	parsnips french fries white potatoes pumpkin	white rice rice cakes	

STEPHANIE'S STORY

"Call me naïve," says Stephanie, "but I didn't know there was something terribly wrong about going six months without menstruating."

Twenty years old and in her last year of university, Stephanie's health was far from superb, but she certainly didn't think that there was anything seriously wrong. A friend suggested she get herself checked out, and she was surprised when the doctor referred her to an OB-GYN for further testing. A few blood tests and an examination later, she had an answer for what was going on in her body. She had polycystic ovarian syndrome.

"The day that she gave me the news, my OB-GYN oh-so-graciously informed me that I would be on medication for the rest of my life, and would most likely be unable to have children, or at least not without fertility treatments. And, oh yes, one more thing … there is nothing you can do about it."

"I'm sure she had no idea, but she had just told me exactly what I needed to hear. At the tender age of 20, with a heart full of dreams for the rest of my life, those words only spurred me on to find out exactly what I could do about it."

Stephanie began to study the way her body worked and what it needed. She discovered her body was craving nutrients it could not get from processed foods. She needed to ditch the industrial convenience and comfort foods, and learn to eat whole, real foods full of nutrients that would nourish her body and ensure that it had what it needed to function well.

She began by slowly making these changes over the course of several years. It wasn't overnight, and it wasn't always easy, but she noticed small improvements within a short period of time, and BIG changes over several years. Her cycle returned and she began ovulating again. Mood swings and sugar cravings decreased, acne improved, and her blood sugar balanced out. "The 5 to 10 extra kilos that I carried simply dropped off, never to come back."

> ## STEPHANIE'S STORY cont'd
>
> "And yes," says Stephanie, "I did get pregnant, all by myself – well, my husband might have played a role." In fact, she went on to have three healthy babies.

Eat alkaline foods

The theory is that a high-acid diet creates a breeding ground for disease and leads to poor health. If you're getting aching joints, gaining weight, craving carbs or sugar, or you have brain fog, then you're running too acidic as I was.

The alkaline diet is 'the opposite' of a typical Western diet. It's based on the idea that optimal health comes from balancing the body's pH by eating more fresh veg and fruit, as well as certain legumes, grains and nuts.

The benefits for PCOS:

1. Promotes fertility. A more alkaline food plan means more alkaline cervical mucus. Since acidic mucous kills sperm, a more alkaline body facilitates the entry of sperm to the uterus and thus improves fertility.
2. Protects your body from a loss of calcium, and so can lead to strong bones and pearly whites.
3. It has been spouted as a great secret to healthy and glowing skin.
4. It can prevent/reduce aches and pains.
5. It will reduce inflammation, and boost your energy and your overall vitality.

Due to eating an acidic diet, women with PCOS are more likely to develop a fatty liver. It is recommended to eat a ketogenic food plan (low-GI carb/higher protein), which improves fatty liver. Once your liver can work well again, your weight loss will speed up! But you must remember to keep the protein healthy and eat the proteins that are right for you, and still include lots of leafy greens. This is important in maintaining an alkaline state.

3. Avoid toxic foods

While you are eating real food, it's just as important to avoid the poisons in our typical Western diet. These are the foods that threw your body out of whack in the first place, so avoid them like the plague. They cause inflammation, thyroid problems, and overproduction of insulin—all of which contribute to hormone imbalance. Some cause your organs considerable stress, which also taxes your hormone balance.

Avoid sugar

Sugar is probably *the biggest culprit* of hormonal imbalances. One can of soft drink contains enough sugar for one week, yet some of us think nothing of drinking one or two cans a day in addition to all the other sugar we systematically consume in our cereals, coffee, condiments and desserts.

Sugar throws your hormones into chaos. First, it prompts your body to produce insulin. There's nothing wrong with insulin, in modest quantities. But when your body produces huge amounts of insulin to deal with too much sugar, the insulin shoots up your testosterone to dangerous levels.

Cravings for sugary foods are actually your body's way of saying it needs to be refuelled. Over the years, we get used to satisfying that craving with manufactured sugar. The craving may be satisfied immediately but the real need is not. For example, when you are hungry and you see a chocolate bar, you may think that you are craving a chocolate bar. That is actually not true. In fact, your body is craving an injection of nutrients and you have trained yourself to fill that craving with a substitute.

In doing so, your digestive system has lost its ability to convert real foods quickly into glucose that goes to your brain and energizes you. You can re-train it. After a few weeks or even days, your body will be able to get as much of a boost from an apple as you used to get from a candy bar.

You will also notice that your body feels more satisfied when you decrease your sugar intake. Sweets and soda taste good but contain no useful nutrients, so you will feel hungry after consuming them. Real food helps to regulate your appetite so you do not overeat.

Avoid table sugar, brown sugar, cane sugar, organic sugar, molasses, maple syrup, and yes, honey. Stop drinking soda.

Avoid processed foods

If you are going to recover from PCOS, you need to cut processed foods out of your diet *entirely*. While real food comes out of the ground and off a tree, processed foods are found in boxes, bags and bottles.

Flour, bread, crackers and pasta are the leading culprits, but they are not the only ones. Some oils, manufactured condiments, deep fried foods, and food that already has the nutrients cooked out of it are all toxic to the human body. Even a glass of orange juice or a bowl of granola can be toxic. Even if it is not from concentrate, the juice is processed from dozens of oranges, which overloads your body with too much fructose in one sitting. The granola is laced with processed sugars.

Any food taken from its original state and broken down into flours, juices, pastes and oils is "processed." It is a recent invention in the history of the human digestive system. The human digestive system is built to process food, not to digest food that has already been processed for us.

We can tolerate an occasional bit of processed food, but cannot deal with it as the main source of our energy. Yet processed foods have become a staple of the Western diet. In the course of your lifetime, odds are you have barely prepared a single meal, or ordered a single meal at a restaurant, that did not have a sizeable portion of bread, pasta, crackers, deep fried foods, white rice or other processed food.

Avoid gluten

Gluten is the major protein in wheat, the most common staple of the Western diet. Contained in breads, crackers, pasta and beer, it's also a main ingredient in boxed cereals, soy sauce, some soups, some potato chips, lollies of all sorts, biscuits, and every wheat-based pastry known to man. Everywhere you find processed food, chances are 'wheat', and therefore gluten, will be in there somewhere.

Gluten plays havoc with the human body. It sits there in your gut creating mischief, creates inflammation and may leak contents into the bloodstream which may cause the so-called beer belly in men and obesity in women. And it contributes to a hormone imbalance as well.

'Gluten-free', by the way, is not a solution. A food that contains no gluten may also contain no nutrients whatsoever, and may have a high glycaemic index. It may also contain loads of refined sugar and who knows what else.

At first, it's hard to resist bread when it's offered at virtually every meal around you. But a funny thing happens when you stop eating it. Not only do you lose the addiction to the taste and texture, it can also become repulsive. You will find your gut gearing up to fight when you smell or see it. It's the same thing that happens to smokers when they quit: the smell of cigarettes can make them nauseous.

CINDY'S SUCCESS STORY

Cindy LOVED bread. Dinner buns, multigrain toast, pizza, specialty crackers, naan bread, English muffins, cranberry muffins, bagels, croissants, tarts, blueberry waffles, lemon cake, pies, biscuits, hamburgers, submarine sandwiches and donuts were all part of her regular fare.

After developing PCOS, she studied the effect of wheat flour and gluten and agreed to go cold turkey and abandon her beloved wheat. The impact was almost instant. Within two days she was feeling more energetic. With a healthy diet of fresh vegetables and real food, she purged the stored junk in her system, and lost 15 kilos in 3 months.

From time to time she indulges in a few bites, but the addiction to wheat has never returned.

Avoid dairy

Milk is good for you, right? No, it's not especially for the majority of the population and according to our blood type diets it contributes to bloating, inflammation, digestive problems, high insulin production, and an underactive thyroid. Too much insulin plus thyroid problems will throw your hormones off balance. Switch to almond milk instead of regular cows' milk.

LAURIE'S SUCCESS STORY

At 26, Laurie's face was full of acne, she was about 10 kilos overweight, and she was experiencing chronic digestive issues. She always felt bloated, and meals made her feel uncomfortable rather than energized. She was drinking at least two glasses of milk a day, and her aesthetician suggested she boycott dairy. She followed the advice. In two weeks, Laurie's face completely cleared. Her digestive issues evaporated, and she lost 12 pounds in two weeks, going down to her normal weight. Today, 26 years later, she has never returned to milk. She enjoys a little cream with her coffee, very small amounts of butter, the occasional ice cream in the summer, and frequent dishes of plain yogurt. The acne, digestive issues, and weight problems never recurred.

Avoid soy and soy products

Soy milk and tofu are good for you, right? Not if you have thyroid issues or hormonal imbalances! Soy contains very high amounts of phytoestrogen or "fake" estrogen as discussed on a few pages ahead, a chemical that resembles estrogen. Some women respond by reducing estrogen production, while other women respond by producing extremely high levels of estrogen. In all cases, regular ingestion of soy harms your hormonal balance and confuses your system. I do believe eating soy was a major cause of my hormone imbalance. If you need to eat tofu and soy, please do it sparingly as most soy products are genetically modified which means bad news for your hormones and body!

Avoid bad fats

Good fats are essential to a healthy diet and promote weight loss. Among other things, they transport water to your skin and other organs, keeping your whole body hydrated. Bad fats cause inflammation and put you at risk of other diseases. When you get bloated and your body stores too much fat, you also produce too much insulin. Bad fats include many oils that are staples in processed foods and deep fried foods— these include vegetable oils such as rapeseed (canola oil) soybean (soybean oil), corn, sunflower, safflower, etc. They were practically non-existent in our diets until the early 1900s when new chemical processes allowed them to be extracted. These different oils contain very large amounts of biologically active fats called Omega-6 poly-unsaturated fatty acids, which are harmful in excess and cause inflammation in the body.

Eat good fats for weight loss and good health—they will be your best friend. Organic butter is actually okay in small quantities—a tablespoon a day. Olive oil, coconut oil and avocado oil are very good for you if you want to lose the weight. Every day I include a scoop of coconut oil in my yummy green smoothie—it fills me up and there is no taste! Give it a go!

Avoid alcohol or limit it

Your digestive system goes into overdrive when you consume alcohol. It acts like you might act if a famous celebrity knocked on your door and offered you a VIP pass to backstage after a concert. It forgets about everything else and uses all its energy to metabolize the alcohol. The real food—including even the sugar within the alcohol—gets stored as fat. It raises your insulin levels in other ways: you tend to make poor food choices when you are tipsy, and you also don't sleep well. Good sleep is a big factor in regulating your insulin levels.

A little wine with dinner is a good choice. But stay away from beer. It is full of gluten and sugar, and is very inflammatory.

Avoid plastic and canned foods

Plastic water bottles and aluminum cans contain a toxin called BPA—bisphenol A. BPA seems to drastically decrease women's production of estrogen and men's production of testosterone. If you have PCOS, chances are you will have much higher levels of BPA in your blood than healthy women.

You will reduce these levels if you eat healthily and stay away from containers that are lined with BPA. If you do find yourself having to use them, do NOT put the plastic in a microwave, leave your water bottle in the sun or heat them up in any way.

Avoid the contraceptive pill

Let's delve into something sensitive… Once upon a time and for longer than 5 years I had taken the pill believing it was the magic answer to help clear my skin and correct my hormonal imbalances.

Firstly, there's no judgment on my behalf whether you choose to take the pill to clear your skin, balance hormones or other-wise. If it works for you and you're happy about it, that's great. But the pill isn't a permanent solution to hormonal problems. At the end of the day it is just a band aid that covers your prob-lems up, and it comes with its drawbacks. And here is the real issue. You can't stay on the pill forever. There will come a time when you're either fed up with the side effects, want to heal the underlying problem, have simply decided that you've been on it too long, or you want to have a baby.

The pill suppresses the body's own ability to make its own hormones. Often after you quit, your body may not be making much progesterone.. It also drastically depletes your Vitamin B6, which you need to make progesterone.

When I came off the pill in 2013, my skin broke out terribly. I was experiencing the repercussions of my body finally having to start producing its own hormones again. I did make use of natural progesterone cream (which I explain later) and supplemented with B6. I suggest you do the same if you want to start to wean yourself off this medication for good.

Be brave and start learning about your hormones, why they may be imbalanced, and how they work. You can do this by learning a bit of hormone knowledge from this book. You'll have such sense of power when you know what's happening within your own body.

Avoid estrogen mimickers

One of the biggest sources of estrogen issues seen in women with PCOS, is due to the substances found in our environment. These substances mimic your own natural estrogen hormone by going into your estrogen receptors and dominating your own natural estrogen, then go on to wreak hormonal havoc in your body. As for the estrogens that are not removed efficiently by your liver's detox pathways, the excess gets stored in fat cells, which means you might end up with fat that you can't seem to get rid of (particularly around the belly - even if you're otherwise skinny!).

In times of stress, malnutrition, pregnancy, rapid weight loss, or otherwise, fat reserves can be mobilized, essentially releasing all these toxic estrogens into your bloodstream. This may result in one or more estrogen related conditions.

There are two classes of estrogen mimickers.

1. Xenoestrogens - these are chemicals that are very similar to estrogens. Most of them are very strong and aggressive, beating the good estrogens to the receptors every time. What's scary is that they are in everything from your makeup to your birth control to your water bottle.

2. Phytoestrogens - these are natural estrogen mimickers found in foods such as soy and flax. They are much weaker than xeno and synthetic estrogens. Some people say they can be helpful to consume because they can compete with the stronger xenoestrogens for the receptors. Others say if you are estrogen dominant, it's not a good idea to consume these kinds of foods. I don't know which is true, but I would be on the side of caution and mostly avoid them as I do now.

Please watch out for a lot of protein shakes that have "soy protein". I was having a soy protein daily leading up to the day I got terribly sick in September 2013. I believe it isn't a coincidence it that my body's hormones were completely messed up after living on soy. To combat this issue, I speak of using DIM supplements which helped correct my estrogen imbalance. You can read about this in the next section.

4. Supplement your diet

In addition to eating real food and avoiding toxic foods, herbs and supplements can help you boost your fertility. They will never replace your nutritional and lifestyle changes, but they can complement and accelerate their impact on your hormones.

Women with PCOS tend to be deficient in a number of key vitamins and other nutrients. So, make sure you are getting enough inositol and folic acid, omega-3 and vitamin D as a start.

When searching for vitamins, please make sure they are *pharmaceutical grade*. Most vitamins on the market are made to a 'food grade level'. Think how a pizza is made—not all pizzas are made with the same quality and quantity of ingredients, right? Well, the same goes with how vitamins are produced. Many studies have tested the ingredients of well-known vitamin brands and most failed by 50%. Many vital ingredients were missing. Let's not mention the absorption levels or lack of with vitamins! This is why most doctors do not believe in vitamins; they consider it to be expensive pee water because the absorption levels are not there. This is all it's worth if your vitamins are not absorbed.

Here is a guide for herbs and supplements to address both your symptoms and the sources of your hormonal imbalances.

Please remember... the goal is not to take 200 pills everyday. I fell into that trap when I first started because I thought every single supplement could help me! Vitamins will never hurt you, however you could be overworking your liver with extra substances (especially if they you are using low quality synthetic vitamins). Also our bodies can only absorb so many nutrients at a time.

Have a look at your test results and see what the major issue in your body is. In my experience and for most women with PCOS require a pharmaceutical grade multivitamin, Omega 3 (to help with the inflammation), a few hormonal balancing supplements such as Vitex and Maca powder and to use DIM to remove excess estrogens in the body. Please note if your liver test comes back and it shows you have a "weak liver", then using DIM can make you break out. My liver could not support detoxification of toxins in my body, so the next place to get rid of them was my skin!

Online supplement shop

You can find all these supplements on the next page online via: www.healmypcos.com/shop to start healing yourself today. Heal My PCOS hampers will also feature, with all the products I used to reduce my inflammation, rebalance hormones, stop the acne and to lose weight.

General supplements required

Please see the tables on the following pages:

General supplements required	
Adaptogen herbs	Adaptogen herbs are important because they help normalise your body's functions – especially those of the endocrine system. They can help reduce feelings of anxiety, and can support healing of your adrenal glands (stress glands). They are non-toxic, nutritive and are safe to use over the long term. Please go to your health food shop to obtain these.
Whole-food multivita-mins	Making sure your body has all of the nutrients necessary is a lot easier when you are taking a whole food multivitamin. Synthetic multivitamins won't have the same effect. Even better, find a whole-food prenatal multivitamin to help prepare the lining of your uterus for childbearing. Please make sure they are pharmaceutical grade too!
Chromium	This trace mineral enhances the action of insulin and may help control blood sugar. In one study women with polycystic ovarian syndrome were given 1000 mcg per day of chromium for two months. Results showed improved insulin sensitivity of 30% to 38%.
Vitamin D	Vitamin D plays an important role in glucose metabolism. It can also restore menstrual regularity in a remarkably short time. You can purchase vitamin D in pill form, (makes sure it is a pharmaceutical grade vitamin however) or you can produce it yourself for free by sitting in the sun for 15 to 20 minutes per day. As long as you do not use sun block, your skin produces vitamin D3 that is then transformed into 10,000 to 25,000 IU of Vitamin D by the kidneys and the liver.

General supplements required	
Calcium	Among many other things, calcium protects cardiovascular health and has a calming effect on your brain and digestive system. Use it with vitamin D to restore menstrual regularity.
Vitamin B complex	Among other things, B vitamins help control your metabolism and blood sugar levels. They also help your liver and thyroid function properly.
To restore hormonal balance	
Omega blend	A blend of omegas is a blend of essential fatty acids (EFAs). EFAs help you lose weight, produce balanced hormones, and nurture a healthy environment for conception. They have been shown to support hormonal balance and production. The correct ratio is (2:omega 3, 1: omega 6, 1: omega 9).
Licorice root (glycyrrhiza glabra)	Helps maintain proper hormone production and release. Supports healthy insulin levels and liver health, which helps restore hormonal balance.
White peony (paeonia lactiflora)	Most clinical trials have found that when White Peony is combined with licorice root it performs better, especially for relaxing muscles and reducing painful menstruation, as well as lowering serum and free testosterone levels in women with PCOS.
Maca (lepidium meyenii)	Maca works to balance the estrogen and progesterone in your body for a healthy menstrual cycle. Maca is an adaptogen and a fertility superfood. By nourishing and balancing the endocrine system, it helps balance the hormones. You can find this at health food shops in a powder form.

To restore hormonal balance	
Vitex (vitex agnus-cas-tus)	Also known as Chaste Tree Berry. Vitex is one of the most powerful herbs for women's fertility and menstrual health, especially if you are not ovulating. By working on the hypothalamic-pituitary-ovarian axis (the hormonal feedback loop), Vitex corrects hormonal imbalances at the source.
Tribulus (tribulus terrestris)	If you use it before ovulation, this wonderful herb may normalise ovulation in infertile women and may improve the timing of your entire menstrual cycle. In fact, Tribulus has been found to be a nourishing tonic for the whole female reproductive system, especially the ovaries.
Natural progesterone cream	Progesterone cream can help oppose the estrogen dominance that occurs with PCOS. By using progesterone cream you can mimic a natural cycle and help the body restore its own cycle, including ovulating. In my research with using bio identical progesterone cream, changes towards a PCOS specific diet and exercise, PCOS could become obsolete. You can purchase natural progesterone cream online via **www.healmypcos.com/shop**. I highly recommend it.
Spearmint/ Peppermint tea	Drink spearmint or peppermint tea and your testosterone levels will plummet. This will help you eliminate acne and male-pattern hair growth.

To restore hormonal balance	
Milk thistle (silybum marianum)	One of your liver's jobs is to purge old hormones out of the bloodstream, and milk thistle is among the most effective remedies for your liver. It helps protect liver cells against damage and promotes healing.
To restore estrogen metabolism	
DIM (Diindolyl-methane)	DIM balances your hormones and helps your system remove excess estrogen. Too much estrogen is a major culprit in many of the fertility issues women face today, including PCOS. It can cause menstrual cycle irregularities and even endometrial hyperplasia. Removal of excess estrogen is vital to overall hormonal balance in women with PCOS.
To boost thyroid function	
Iodine	The form of iodine you need varies depending on your constitution and type of thyroid dysfunction. Your naturopath may recommend Edgar Cayce's remedies, which have proven very powerful. You can also get daily iodine from kelp supplements and seaweed.
Selenium	If your thyroid levels are very low, you could be seriously deficient in selenium. You can get selenium as supplements or eat two brazil nuts each day.

For hirsutism and endometrial hyperplasia	
Saw Palmetto (Serenoa repens)	Saw Palmetto has been found to inhibit DHT production by reducing 5 alpha-reductase production, which may help prevent hirsutism in women with PCOS. This herb also helps reduce endometrial hyperplasia and hormonal acne symptoms. Saw palmetto is like the weaker, natural version of the drug Spirolactone (which I was prescribed for my acne) for hormonal acne, except it can come with scary side effects. I suggest give the Saw Palmetto a go first.
To restore healthy insulin function	
Cinnamon	A pilot study published in 2007 by Fertility & Sterility shows that cinnamon greatly reduces insulin resistance in women with PCOS. Another study suggests it may also reduce insulin resistance by slowing the movement of food from the stomach to the small intestine. This slows the breakdown of carbohydrates, which is important for people with diabetes and women with PCOS.
Gymnema (Gymnema sylvestre, G.sylvestris)	Gymnema has been used for hundreds of years to reduce high blood sugar. This herb has a sugar-blocking action on taste buds and the small intestine. It blocks the typical paths that sugar molecules take during digestion, delaying absorption. It helps the pancreas reproduce the cells that produce insulin, which aids in more insulin production, which stimulates the production of enzymes to help with the uptake of glucose into cells, and which then prevents stimulation of the liver to produce more glucose. Gymnema also appears to have a lipid-lowering effect, which aids in weight loss.

To restore healthy insulin function	
Zinc	Zinc is a trace mineral whose deficiency is highly correlated with acne. In addition to balancing your blood sugar levels and acne, zinc also helps your immune and digestive system, and (in cooperation with vitamin A and vitamin E) aids your thyroid function.
Magnesium (powder)	It seems magnesium helps to control insulin levels. Like calcium, it can also have a sedative effect on your blood. When you are stressed, you tend to use up the magnesium in your system, so it is good to take magnesium powder as it is easily absorbable when you are stressed. I took 1 cap full of magnesium in the morning and night when I was full of acne and in pain with my periods and it helped relieved it a lot!
Epsom Salt Bath	The best way to replenish your stores and get your magnesium levels up to scratch is via an Epsom salt bath. When laying in the bath the magnesium gets absorbed into your body. Oral magnesium supplementation can sometimes be poorly absorbed and cause loose stools at far lower doses, meaning it's hard to get enough to get your levels up. Visit our online store to purchase the magnesium salt mix I use for my baths – daily.
Co-enzyme Q10 (CoQ10)	The CoQ10 in your body helps you produce energy and maintain good metabolism. It helps women control blood sugar levels.

To restore healthy insulin function	
Probiotics	Take one probiotic a day to help your digestive system function properly. Gut health is so important. Increasing the bacteria in your stomach and other digestive organs helps you absorb nutrients efficiently and enhances your insulin function.

To control inflammation	
Omega-3s	Omega essential fatty acids, especially omega-3, decrease the risk of inflammation. Western diets are deficient in omega-3 fatty acids, and have excessive amounts of omega-6 fatty acids. Omega-6 is pro-inflammation and omega-3 is anti-inflammation. Studies show human beings evolved on a diet with a ratio of omega-6 to omega-3 essential fatty acids (EFA) of approximately 1 whereas in Western diets the ratio is 15/1-16.7/1. (4) Getting enough essential fatty acids, especially the omega-3, will control inflammation, whether you obtain these through foods you eat or through supplements.
Cod liver oil	An amazing superfood for the liver, hormones and skin is fermented cod liver oil. It's full of good fats, Vitamin A, D, K, and anti-inflammatory Omega 3 and it's helped me with my skin and breakouts.
Systemic enzyme therapy	Systemic enzyme blends modify your biological responses. They work with your body's own immune defense system to moderate the inflammatory response. They also break down the proteins in the blood that cause inflammation.

To control inflammation	
Royal jelly + bee propolis	Both royal jelly and bee propolis have been shown to reduce inflammation and naturally boost the body's immune system. They may also aid in hormonal balance through endocrine system support.
To help with food intolerances	
Digestive Enzyme	Gut health is crucial. Take a digestive enzyme daily to help with the digestion of food and food intolerances.

5. Lifestyle changes

Healing yourself requires commitment, ingenuity, and a change of lifestyle. If you envision it, and plan it, you can do it. Stick to your guns and remember, you are Number One.

Listen to your body

Eat when you get hungry! Nourish yourself when your body tells you to. Do NOT starve yourself.

On the other hand, don't eat if you are not hungry. If it's time for lunch and you feel like you only need a salad, then just eat a salad. If dinnertime comes and you don't feel hungry enough for a meal, wait an hour or two until you do feel hungry. Your body knows best.

It does not matter if you are underweight or overweight. The key is to listen to your body and nourish yourself with real food.

Avoid fast food joints

It is a good idea to avoid eating out for awhile. When you do order meals, it is possible to fully satisfy yourself with real food, but you may need to negotiate with the restaurateur, server, or menu.

Get more sleep

When you have healthy sleep habits, your whole body will feel satisfied and happy. Overnight, your liver goes into high gear, processing toxins, strange chemicals, and even new experiences. It is absolutely crucial for purging toxins, healing, adjusting, and repairing.

When you stay awake past midnight you interfere with the liver's most powerful work. The liver works best in total darkness, so turn off the night light too.

Think of sleep as a big meal. When you don't get enough sleep, your body will crave greater quantities of food. Less sleep also means your body will not burn as much fat.

Your brain will thank you too. Dreams and all kinds of mental organization happen during sleep. It helps you reduce stress.

Check your pH levels

Your pH level is an extremely important tool when checking your health. Your body's pH is measured on a scale of 0 to 14, where neutral pH would be considered 7.

Studies have shown that when your pH level falls below 6.2 it can affect your ability to conceive. As you go lower, your blood would be considered more acidic, while higher would be considered more alkaline.

You can easily test your pH levels at home which I do regularly. Simply go to your local chemist or drug store and ask your pharmacist for a pH kit. While you can't actually control your body's own pH levels, you can help make it easier for your body to do it on your behalf. Keeping yourself healthy with a good diet (sticking to less acidic foods) and minimizing harmful habits is likely going to be more than enough to avoid having your blood pH flagged during your next health professional's appointment.

Drink peppermint tea

If you are suffering from severe acne like I was, then give peppermint tea a go—it really helped me! Remember that high insulin levels cause our ovaries to create more testosterone. The more insulin you have in your body, the more testosterone you have. The more testosterone you have, the more acne you have.

Research suggests that women with PCOS who drank two cups of peppermint tea per day for one month showed much lower testosterone levels than the control group. The study concluded that peppermint tea is a helpful natural treatment for hirsutism and acne in PCOS. I would drink two cups during my recovery and if I ever get any spots on my chin (due to hormones) I will have two cups of peppermint tea and it normally reduced the severity of my breakout.

Give acupuncture a go

Normal acupuncture and electro acupuncture have very been successful in my healing and reducing stress ... even though I'm afraid of needles! Trust me, it doesn't hurt and it is such a relaxing experience. Electro acupuncture involves passing a low-frequency electric pulse through fine wires attached to acupuncture needles.

A study published in the June 2009 issue of American Journal of Physiology-Regulatory, Integrative and Comparative Physiology found a group of women undertaking electro-acupuncture treatments experienced more regular menstrual cycles, reduced testosterone levels and reduced waist circumference. Hallelujah!

Acupuncture helps by treating the root cause of the PCOS—hormonal imbalances. It focuses on balancing and regulating important hormones related to PCOS and will re-establish and increase blood flow and nutrient supply to the uterus and ovaries.

After a month of my own treatment, I noticed I had a regular menstruation and ovulation, and also less pain, less excess hair and less acne! Ring and book in an appointment today and trust me when I say it will not hurt.

Use natural progesterone cream

This step is really important if you believe you'll struggle with the recommended diet, you're overweight, stressed, over the age of 35 and if your cysts fail to respond to diet alone.

Progesterone is the hormone that signals the end of ovulation and causes the remaining follicles to shrink. It is made from fats extracted from wild yams. I do recommend using only a natural progesterone cream, not a synthetic prescribed pill. It can cause so many more problems you don't want to deal with.

The Natural progesterone cream I used contains a straight disogenin from wild yams (from which bio-identical USP progesterone is made) however it is not the same thing. It is similar and may have benefits, but is not quite exactly the same as our body□s progesterone.

The usual dose of progesterone is 20 mg per day, used for 14 days before the first day of your period (days 12 - 26 of your cycle). This simulates your natural cycle, where progesterone climbs during and after ovulation to prepare your body to receive a fertilised egg. When the egg doesn't come, progesterone falls, and menstruation begins. So stopping right before your period will signal for your body to begin menstruating.

The recommended product used in my recovery is called 'Women's Balance' by Kororo. It's made with organic ingredients. You'll need three jars or two pump bottles for eight weeks of use. I recommend you use this for a few months and then wean yourself off it if you have low progesterone from your blood tests. Again, this is just something to aid you whilst your body's hormones are naturally rebalancing.

You can find this product on our online store: www.healmypcos.com/store. Or alternatively Email me if you are interested in the product: info@healmypcos.com

Love your liver

Beyond a healthy lifestyle, one of the first things we want to look at when it comes to hormonal imbalances, is how your liver is functioning. This is because a healthy liver is the key to healthy hormone balance!

Many women with PCOS develop "fatty liver" and it currentlyaffects up to 15% to 55% of women suffers, depending on the diagnostic criteria used.

Fatty liver is said to occur when excess triglycerides (fat) are stored in the liver. This causes inflammation and damage to your liver cells. Put simply, your liver isn't meant to store fat; its role is to be a detox organ for the body filtering out harmful substances.

Your liver is detoxifying all day every day through something called "detoxification pathways", and it performs this in two distinct phases.

In Phase I, called "oxidation", the liver uses oxygen and enzymes to change the hormones and toxins into a more water soluble form so that they can easily be excreted by the kidneys or bowel.

In Phase II, called "conjugation", oxidized chemicals are combined with sulfur, specific amino acids, or organic acids, and then excreted.

My liver was underperforming when I was first diagnosed with PCOS. To this date it is still kind of sluggish, so I've had to learn to love my liver to allow it to perform to release any toxins from my body. Otherwise acne will soon show on my face!

You can check your levels of your liver function tests, or "LFTs" with your health professional.

It is also your role to learn to LOVE YOUR LIVER and help it not hinder it if you want to have good skin, healthy weight and good energy.

Here are some healthy lifestyle changes you can adopt to start loving your liver today:

- Switch the majority of your diet away from processed foods that contain chemicals. Eat good fats, not bad fats.
- Avoid excessive Omega 6 fatty acids (which overwhelms the liver and is inflammatory) and concentrate on Omega 3s (which are extremely anti-inflammatory).

- Change all of your skin care products to natural products, and eliminate those that aren't. Visit our online shop via: www.healmypcos.com/shop to find out which skin care products I use that are great for acne prone skin.

- Watch the environmental toxins in your home - switch to more natural cleaning products, consider safer cookware, and get house plants that filter the stuffy indoor air.

- Minimize the use of caffeine, alcohol, and cigarettes.

- Keep your stress levels in check, as emotional toxins can also lead to an inefficient liver.

- A great supplement for the liver, hormones and skin is fermented cod liver oil. Its full of good fats, Vitamin A, D, K, and anti-inflammatory Omega 3 fatty acids. It can go a long way to relieving monthly breakouts, and I'm not the only one who thinks so. See more about Cod liver oil in the supplement section of this book.

Forget about your weight

Eat healthily, build muscle, and get lots of sleep, and your weight will settle where it wants to. Don't worry about it! Remember, worrying about weight may have gotten you into this rather painful place to start with.

Don't push it!

Let your body heal on its own schedule. It may take weeks or months. There is no deadline.

6. Build some muscle

The best kind of exercise for restoring system balance and optimizing your energy is muscle training. It's tougher than stationary bikes and treadmills but the results are fantastic! You will be truly amazed at what a difference it can mean for your everyday tasks, your energy levels, your appetite, the quality of your sleep, and your state of mind. In fact, muscle training is the best anti-depressant that exists.

Your muscles are sitting there waiting to be used, torn, and rebuilt. They are in your body, not something you have to buy. They are one of the most amazing personal assets you have, and simply by building them, you can rebuild your strength and your whole constitution.

Invest in a personal trainer

For motivational purposes, I strongly recommend you invest in a proven personal trainer, male or female. If you cannot afford one, use this chapter as a guide and find a good trainer on YouTube!

No, you don't have to jog

Jogging and so-called aerobic exercises do not deliver noticeable benefits in return for your time. According to the blood type diets, some people's biochemistry is more inclined to lifting heavy weights for weight loss.

Jogging for five minutes is a warm up, and not the best kind by any means. Read on.

No, you don't need any special equipment! All you need is a rubber mat or yoga mat, a free wall, and some free weights. A bench is a bonus. This means you do NOT need to buy a gym membership or spend any extra money.

No, you won't need to spend an hour! Keep your workouts to 30 minutes. This includes 5 minutes warming up and 5 minutes cooling off and stretching.

Choose an exercise you love. I love walking outside, in the fresh air and listening to my favourite upbeat and enchanting music for 30 minutes a day. Because I love walking, I do it everyday and it is NOT EXERCISE to me. What kind of exercises do you love doing? Make it a habit and enjoy yourself.

Do full-body five-minute warm-ups

Warming up is absolutely essential for successful workouts. Most importantly, it drastically decreases the risk of injury.

All you need is five minutes to warm up your muscles and joints and get your heart rate up. Don't do stretches because they can increase the chance of injury when you are doing muscle workouts.

Two fantastic examples of warm-up exercises can be found at:

www.healmypcos.com/warm-ups

When you do squats, make sure your knees do not protrude past your toes.

Give yourself a few days to get into the swing of these exercises. Refer constantly to the videos to ensure you have the right form.

Get ready to test your muscles!

Muscle training puts your whole body to the test and strength training should be a part of your treatment plan. This is particularly important to women with PCOS because we do suffer from insulin resistance; the inability to properly react to our own insulin.

When you train your muscles to bear weights—even the weight of your body—you are training your heart to pump blood and nutrients to the muscle, and you are training your lungs to send oxygen to the heart.

It takes a while for your organs to learn the new routine, but you're the boss, and they will learn! The result is a far more efficient body. Strength training doesn't just help you get stronger, it increases your muscle mass.

Here are two excellent examples of full-body muscle training. They look simple but they deliver results. They may look easy but you will feel the pain after 10, 15 or 30 repetitions. Keep your muscle training to 20 or 30 minutes max.

www.healmypcos.com/strength-exericses

'Core exercises' work your entire body and heart. They are the most important. When you focus on large muscles such as your thighs, glutes, abs and shoulders, you will see the most results.

You may find lower body exercises easier than those involving your shoulders and arms, but keep in mind women typically have stronger lower bodies and weaker upper bodies, so make sure you do all the upper body exercises.

Does it hurt?

Yes, building muscle hurts in several ways: muscle soreness, nausea, and breathlessness. You will feel pain as you increase repetitions, and as your workout proceeds you will feel your heart working harder. After 20 minutes it may feel like you are about to keel over and die.

Muscle soreness

In order to "build" muscle, you first have to "tear" muscle. It's like an elastic band that you keep snapping. If you snap it often enough, it will break. Unlike an elastic band, however, muscles miraculously rebuild themselves. When they do so, they are bigger and more efficient. The soreness you feel a few hours or a few days after you work a muscle group will become both familiar and comforting to you. It means your muscles have broken and they are "healing" and growing.

You do not want to feel pain or stress on your joints or your spine. Pay very close attention to the form your personal trainer shows you. Get the form down first to prevent injury. You will catch on with practice.

When you first start out, intense strength training involves a sudden increase in lactic acid. It can make you feel like you will pass out or throw up. This will happen only during the first two or three workouts. Prepare a smoothie ahead of time so you can drink it immediately following your workout. Keep water handy and take big gulps when absolutely necessary. Drink a whole glass of water at the end of your workout. The feeling will pass.

Breathlessness

With muscle training, you are training your heart and lungs and blood to be more efficient. Trust me, it works. If you push yourself to finish the repetitions with no break, it can feel like you have no more breath and you are going to die. You won't. It's okay to huff and puff and sweat.

Good workouts include 30-second rests when you are out of breath. Limit it to 30 seconds because you want to keep your heart rate up.

Cool down!

Spend five minutes cooling down and stretching. This helps in several ways. First, it reduces the muscle soreness over the next 24 to 36 hours as your muscles rebuild. Secondly, it will lower cortisol levels (cortisol acts as a fat storage hormone).

I always meditate for 5 minutes after every gym session. People do look at me strangely! I put on a meditation song from my phone and lie down and do deep breathing. However, I feel good knowing I'm lowering my cortisol levels and avoiding adding further stress to my body. Cooling down also prepares you for your next meal.

Eat immediately after your workout

When you eat right away, you are training your system to expect rewards for its work. Your system needs to replenish all the fuel it has exhausted. The nutrients you digest now will be delivered straight to where they are most needed, so all the food will be processed most efficiently.

Then take a nap if you need to.

Give your muscles time to rebuild

Especially during the first few weeks, you will need to give your muscles ample time to heal before you test them again.

If your muscles have not healed yet, they will not be able to carry any weight. Sleep is absolutely crucial to building muscle.

For the first few days and weeks you may find yourself walking funny. The soreness may be intense. Take a hot bath with Epsom salts, and stay mobile, move around. Stick with it!

Real benefits of resistance training

To recap, doing any type of resistance training such as weight lifting training is beneficial and encouraged. It definitely helped with my insulin resistance. Benefits will include:

- Release of hormones that have anti-ageing benefits, including improved skin and a youthful experience
- Excess cortisol (stress hormones) being swept from the bloodstream
- Improved insulin sensitivity because your muscles and cells are desperate for fuel during and after your workout

and will last 24 hours after a workout
- Boosted immunity and an increased sense of well-being
- Improved sleep quality

7. Reduce your stress

With a healthy diet, healthy lifestyle and good workout regimen, you are on your way. But stress can seriously undermine your progress. Among the causes of hormonal imbalance, stress exacerbates any other issues that may cause polycystic ovarian syndrome. Cortisol is secreted when you are physically or mentally stressed, and it increases your insulin levels and testosterone. Over time, it has a devastating impact on your hormones.

Yes, you CAN eliminate stress from your life. If you think your personal circumstances make stress unavoidable, think again. It is possible to live your life without worry or fear, no matter where you are or what your life is like.

Are you stressed out about PCOS?

Even having PCOS can make you feel stressed out. It can challenge your confidence, self-esteem, and feelings of self-worth. You can get worried about losing your boyfriend or husband or partner because you have completely lost all interest in sex. Acne can be painful on your skin, and you may worry what people will think when they see acne on your face.

I don't blame you for feeling anxious about all these things. I can relate! But the stress is actually unnecessary. The thing is, your current situation is a temporary thing. It will pass, and you will live to tell the tale. So settle in, follow your plan, and watch yourself transform before your very eyes. Enjoy the journey as much as the destination.

Stress can be a choice

We are accustomed to blaming our circumstances or other people for the stress we feel. We are taught from a young age to respond to things with worry, dread and anxiety. We are even encouraged to feel anxious about things.

But it's actually our own choice. And there is another way, a way that very few of us have ever been taught. Just as we choose to worry about things, we can choose not to worry about them.

I strongly recommend you read the books on the reading list and learn how to eliminate stress from your life. It works!

Start to meditate

Meditation can be an immense help. It can get you back into the present moment so you stop worrying about life, your diet, your weight etc. It can help you focus on yourself and your body while giving you a sense of calm.

Meditation is a state of thought awareness. It is not an act of doing—it is a state of awareness. True meditation is a profound, deep peace that occurs when the mind is calm, yet silent and still completely alert. Meditation is seen by a number of researchers as potentially the most effective form of stress reduction.

I was scared to start meditating. I thought only people on top of mountains ever meditated ... haha! It's been so beneficial in my recovery. I meditate for at least 30 minutes every morning before I start my day.

How do you start to meditate?

Set aside 10-30 minutes per day. Some people find that beginning the day in a state of peace and silence makes the whole day better. Others find the evening is best, where the soothing effects help take them into deep and nourishing sleep. I tend to do meditation at night before I go to sleep or after a gym workout. I have friends who do it during their workday at work! It's a satisfying feeling once you finish.

YouTube is a great place to start searching for meditations. I recommend 'Guided Meditations' or 'Open Heart Meditations'. I personally use a mobile app called 'Simply Being' from iTunes and it works wonders! They have a large list of amazing calming meditations to choose from. I love zoning out and feeling connected. I encourage you to schedule it in EVERY DAY as part of your recovery.

Pursue laughter

When was the last time you experienced a full belly laugh? The kind where you are doubled over, red-faced, holding your gut? The kind that makes your belly muscles sore afterward?

This is the laughter that heals. When you laugh, you cannot feel any worry, stress, sadness or anything negative. It releases you—catapults you—from any form of doubt or fear. It brings you back into the present moment where there is no regret about a past and no worry for a future.

Pursue the company of people who make you laugh. Watch funny movies and stand-up comedy. Hang around kids and act silly.

Release your tears

Tears are a crucial method your body uses to purge itself and heal. Let them flow, even if you have to sob. Often laughter helps you liberate your tears, and it's perfectly fine when the two of them happen at once!

After a good cry, hydrate yourself with a glass of water, a cup of herbal tea, and a hot bath. All the better if you have a good meal too!

Let your workouts release your stress

Strength training and intense workouts are among the best stress-busters on the planet. Enjoy building muscle and watch the stress fall away!

8. Read some good books

Good books will not just inform and enlighten you. They will empower you. Here are some quality additions to your library. You can buy used copies in great condition for bargain prices on Amazon, Bookdepository, Booktopia or your local bookstore.

Self-love books

The Gifts of Imperfection, by Brene Brown

This is my favourite. When I had a meltdown after breaking up with the person I thought I would marry in 2011, a dear friend told me about this book. It started my whole journey of self-discovery, self-love and self-care. Let go of who you think you're supposed to be, says Brown, and embrace who you are. What a way to start your new life! You will feel weights falling off your shoulders just after reading it!

Loving What Is, by Byron Katie

This book gave me so many ah-ha moments. It caused me to reflect on all my actions and start realising my words and everything in life may just be a reflection of my inner thoughts. If you ever wanted to release anger, resentment, jealousy, hatred, stress, worry or bitterness, Byron Katie will show you how easy it is! This book can truly change your life, as it has mine.

The Power of Intention, by Wayne Dyer

Another great read that has had a massive impact on my life. Do you find yourself feeling bad for people who are in a tough situation? Do you worry about other people all the time? Wayne Dyer shows how utterly futile that behaviour is. Choose to feel good, he says, and watch what happens!

You Can Heal Your Life, by Louise Hay

Wow. This book is a MUST. This made me realise the power of emotions and how they can truly affect your health. This self-help classic has been translated into 29 languages since it was first published in 1984, and has sold more than 35 million copies in over 35 countries. Hold it close to your heart as you take charge of your own health.

The Power is Within You, by Louise Hay

This book captivated me. Louise Hay has been a massive support in my recovery. Did you know at only 22 years of age, Louise Hay healed herself of vaginal cancer? How did she do it? She changed the way she thought about her past, and changed her present choices. The cancer vanished and never returned. Louise is now in her 80s and one of the world's most beloved spiritual leaders. In this book she shares powerful secrets of mental and physical health.

Wheat Belly, by William Davis

If you think going off bread and wheat-based products can be tougher than quitting cigarettes, this book will make it easier for you. Learn how wheat products have become the single biggest dietary factor that contributes to the epidemic of obesity and fatal diseases in the Western world.

In an Unspoken Voice, by Dr Peter Levine

If you, like many human beings on the planet, suffered abuse in your childhood or teens, your body still carries residual reflexes from the incidents. The subtitle for the book is 'How the body releases trauma and restores goodness', and Dr Levine shows how you can do this. A very fascinating study!

Health books + films + documentaries

Food Matters™ by James Colquhoun and Laurentine Ten Bosch

Food Matters – Wow. What can I say? I get chills every time I watch this short film. It provides a radiant beacon of hope with steps you can do today to take control of your health. Anyone who is serious about their health and wants to take steps towards healing PCOS and any health issues needs to see this stunning film.

Register to watch the first 40 minutes of the film here: http://www.foodmatters.tv/

Hungry for Change film by James Colquhoun and Laurentine ten Bosch

Being someone who use to drink four cans of 'diet coke' per day and—I hate to admit it—lived on diet pills to lose weight, this movie really opened my eyes! It's the latest Food Matters film and exposes shocking secrets the diet, weight loss and food industry don't want you to know about. This exposé of their deceptive strategies, designed to keep you craving more and more, was an eye opener. Could the foods we are eating actually be keeping us stuck in the diet trap?

See the preview here: https://youtu.be/3MvAM97VDE8

Register to watch the first 40 minutes of the documentary here: http://www.hungryforchange.tv/

Sugar the Bitter Truth by Norman W. Walker

I watched this documentary in February 2013. It opened my eyes to the damaging effects of sugary diet. It's an hour long, so make yourself a nice green tea and sit back and relax and enjoy. They argue that fructose (too much) and fibre (not enough) appear to be cornerstones of the obesity epidemic through their effects on insulin.

See the documentary here: https://youtu.be/dBnni-ua6-oM

Real Food Kitchen book by Dr Libby Weaver

This is one of my favourite cookbooks of all time. Dr Libby has a PhD in studying the human body and cells. Her cookbook is your answer to preparing and eating healthy, delicious, family friendly meals that light up your soul and your energy. You can buy her book online: www.drlibby.com

9. Now it's up to you

With my final words, I want to remind you to have patience.

Depending on the severity of your hormonal imbalance, it could take a while to heal. If you can learn from this book and put my advice into practice on a day to day basis, you can heal yourself from polycystic ovarian syndrome. You can rebalance your hormones, get back your menstrual cycle, feel sexy again, and bear children.

The goal with this book is to give you the knowledge to learn how to heal yourself forever and you will. When you know where your most pressing health issues are, you can take the steps laid out in my book to overcome these issues through simple lifestyle changes.

 I hope this book gives you the knowledge you need to act as your own advocate, and the power to create change in your life ... starting today. Many women have healed naturally, including me and you can too.

I want to hear from you.

Please get in touch with me and share your success story.

Send an email to: info@healmypcos.com

Thank you for reading. I wish you all the best in your healing months moving forward.

Keep smiling ;)

Lots of love

Melissa xoxo

About the author

Melissa Madgwick is a a real 31 year old woman who is on the other side of healing from polycystic ovarian syndrome – naturally. She was a professional dancer in ballet, tap and jazz for 15 years. She is a certified health and food coach, has a university degree and is a passionate entrepreneur. Life shifted when Melissa took her health into her own hands three years ago. For 10 years, her "normal adult life" consisted of terrible acne breakouts lasting three months at a time, terrible menstrual pains and heavy bleeding, fluctuating weight, zero sex drive, horribly moody and an under-active thyroid function.

Melissa's life now revolves around natural living and healing. She is an avid health advocate who specialises in working with women who are suffering from PCOS. Now feeling the best Melissa has in years, she eagerly helps other women overcome the PCOS dis-ease holistically. Her heart signs when hearing success stories from the simple shifts in diet, mindset and lifestyle. Melissa looks forward to sharing her healing journey with you. You can follow Melissa and join the Heal My PCOS tribe via: www.healmypcos.com.

CPSIA information can be obtained
at www.ICGtesting.com
Printed in the USA
LVHW010918050119
602872LV00041B/1873/P

9 780994 540461